INTEGRATING PERSPECTIVES ON HEALTH

Edited by
Neil Cooper, Chris Stevenson and Glynis Hale

Open University Press
Buckingham · Philadelphia

Open University Press
Celtic Court
22 Ballmoor
Buckingham
MK18 1XW

and

1900 Frost Road, Suite 101
Bristol, PA 19007, USA

First Published 1996

A catalogue record of this book is available from the British Library

ISBN   0 335 19356 0 (pb)   0 335 19357 9 (hb)

Library of Congress Cataloging-in-Publication Data
Integrating perspectives on health / Neil Cooper, Chris Stevenson,
    and Glynis Hale.
        p.   cm.
    Includes bibliographical references and index.
    ISBN 0-335-19357-9 (hardcover). – ISBN 0-335-19356-0 (pbk.)
    1. Social medicine. 2. Medicine and psychology. 3. Health.
  4. Nursing–Social aspects. I. Cooper, Neil, 1961–
  II. Stevenson, Chris, 1953– . III. Hale, Glynis, 1957– .
  RA418.I523 1996
  610–dc20   95–47214
                                                            CIP

Typeset by Dorwyn Ltd, Rowlands Castle, Hants
Printed in Great Britain by St Emundsbury Press Ltd, Bury St Edmunds, Suffolk

Contents

To the health studies students who asked the challenging questions which helped to bring the book into existence.

Notes on contributors

Phil Barker is professor of psychiatric nursing practice at the University of Newcastle. His special interests are in alternative paradigms in nursing research inquiry, interdisciplinary collaboration, and social and cultural differences in concepts of health and illness.

Neil Cooper is a lecturer in health studies at the University of Sunderland. After working as a staff nurse in child development, he became increasingly interested in the social sciences and read anthropology and psychology at the University of London. As a research assistant he developed an interest in child abuse and child protection, and his academic interests now lie in lay-professional discourse within the child protection field.

Stewart Forster graduated in psychology and philosophy from Sunderland Polytechnic in 1991. He completed nurse training (adult) at Newcastle College of Health Studies in 1995, and is currently working as a staff nurse in neurological medicine at the Royal Victoria Infirmary, Newcastle.

John Fulton was head of post-registration education and training for nurses at Bede College of Health Studies before taking up his current position as principal lecturer in health and nursing studies at the University of Sunderland. His research interests centre on nurses' constructions of their caring experience.

Richard Gamlin has a senior lectureship at the University of Northumbria at Newcastle, supported by Marie Curie Cancer Care. He has extensive experience of hospice work and works in partnership with Shaun Kinghorn.

Glynis Hale became disenchanted with her work as a radiographer and studied psychology and religion at the University of Sunderland. Her PhD thesis focused on the social construction of death and bereavement, and she retains a research interest in this area. She has also developed a practice side to this area through counselling.

Shaun Kinghorn has several years' experience in oncology nursing and palliative care and currently works alongside Richard Gamlin at the University of Northumbria as a lecturer in cancer/palliative case studies.

Alison McInnes is a lecturer in health studies and social work at the University of Sunderland. She is a qualified social worker with special interests in drug use, older people and child protection issues.

Pauline Pearson is a health visitor and lecturer in primary care nursing at Newcastle University. She has worked in a variety of health visiting posts in inner-city and suburban areas. She now works mainly in research, where her interests include consumer perceptions, multidisciplinary working and the interface between primary and secondary care.

Chris Stevenson has a professional background in community psychiatric nursing and is currently a lecturer in psychiatric nursing practice at the University of Newcastle. Prior to this, she lectured in health studies at the University of Sunderland. Her PhD work was in family therapy, looking particularly at how the differing world-views of participants require negotiation towards a therapeutic context.

Nigel Watson presently teaches health promotion and the sociology of health at the University of Sunderland. He has worked in the field as a health promotion practitioner, most recently with responsibility for community development initiatives. His research interests focus around issues of participation in health-enhancing processes and the social construction of 'normal' health.

Acknowledgements

The book was produced with the support of many people, both direct and indirect. Our families and friends were not merely tolerant, but often actively involved in offering ideas when our scholarly pursuits became entangled in paradoxes which mirrored the field being explored. Especial thanks go to Catherine for her (non-formally attributed) 'contribution'.

We are grateful for the helpful comments on Chapter 11 provided by Dr Irene Whitehill; to Wendy Stainton Rogers who first questioned the sense of integrating perspectives into a 'tidy' model; to an Australian visitor, Cheryl Waters, who hinted that our ideas of what constituted a discipline could be broader.

We are also indebted to our colleagues at Sunderland, especially David Blackwell and Keith Holden, for raising problems when we thought all was going smoothly.

Preface

All three of the editors, and some of the other contributors, have taught aspects of health studies to students at the University of Sunderland. We have sat and talked to individual students about academic understandings of health. We have discussed health-related issues in seminars, and confidently lectured to students about how health may be understood through combining the respective knowledges of biology, psychology and sociology. Students appear to grasp what the different understandings of health mean in their acceptance of a biopsychosocial model of health. But the different understandings based upon biological, psychological and social knowledge about health and illness rest as uneasy allies. The tensions which operate between these three different types of knowledge are largely ignored, and it seemed that these tensions could form the focus of a book. We felt that the tensions could be explored and an attempt made at a reconciliation to facilitate students in developing an integrated understanding of health. This was the idea, but as Feyerabend (1991: 163) suggested, '. . . ideas like butterflies, do not really exist; they develop, they enter into relations with other ideas and they have effects'. As we attempted to articulate our concerns and consider what the biopsychosocial model actually was and where it had originated, and how practice and understandings of health may be limited by it, both interconnections and confusions were created. The book is not a finished text, but a place where the butterfly has rested for a brief moment before taking once more to its uncertain flight.

Originally, when we decided to edit a book about perspectives on health, our thoughts turned to the contribution that our many colleagues and acquaintances with clinical experience could make. The editors would cleverly draw together the clinicians' ideas into an integrated model of health, justifying the title. Our aim was deeply naive on two counts. First, we had assumed that integration was desirable. This was probably driven by our own perceived needs as teachers. The book was precipitated by the needs expressed by health studies students, who were struggling to construct integrated accounts of health and illness. Their challenge was to find accounts which were consistent with the generic perspective taken within their degree programme, while assimilating knowledge from disciplines which are underpinned by very different forms of explanation. We also were driven by the desire to justify health studies as a discipline in its own right, and felt that a more coherent model would be critical in achieving this end.

Second, we had assumed that integration was possible. As editors, we simply had to find the right 'key'. At the end of our writing and editing, we are less confident (?arrogant) that a neat solution is possible. In some ways, we think that a degree of diversity of explanation is to be celebrated, and that homogenization is less attractive. Although the title remains the same, the stance taken to integration has changed. We now see the book as an attempt to provide some narratives concerning the tensions and possibilities when different views of health and illness are considered. We then take these narratives as a starting point for discourse between those who study, research and practise in the area.

1

The biopsychosocial model

Neil Cooper, Chris Stevenson and Glynis Hale

Introduction

This chapter outlines the biopsychosocial model in the context of a rising critique of the medical model from academics, and from the development of health and social care professions such as nursing and social work. The recognition of medicine's failure to 'cure' common chronic diseases, and its inability to respond to general societal changes, has also meant a challenge to its status.

First, the biopsychosocial model will be considered. It is suggested that the model has emerged as a nominal description of explanations in health. It will then be argued that the alignment of disciplinary knowledge within the model is not an integrated form but an uneasy association of explanations which are both hierarchically organized and contain the inherent potential for conflict and confusion. These conflicts and confusions are not adequately addressed, despite the model being used extensively in practice.

It will be demonstrated that the medical model, which is perceived to be a unified theoretical entity, has adapted to changing social and cultural circumstances, and that the medical model as we know it is a relatively recent phenomenon. In the context of this chapter and the book as a whole, the medical model is defined as a label referring to practices based upon the concept that health problems have specific causes which can be identified, and that, because of the identification, cure is possible with the removal of the root cause. The evolution of the critiques against the medical model, and the medical practices derived from it, will demonstrate how challenges to the medical model created the impetus for the development of a biopsychosocial model. The maturing of other professions such as nursing and social work will be examined, and it will be shown that the professionalization of these occupations with the identification of discrete bodies of knowledge and models of practice challenged the medical model. Medicine's failure to cure chronic conditions such as heart disease and cancer will be considered in relation to emerging fields of health promotion, response to death and dying, and the value of complementary medicines.

While the developments and actions discussed in this chapter are not linear in movement but progress with constant dynamic feedback, the writing of a book chapter forces some form of linear construction of the story. It is important to remember that many events were occurring simultaneously and developments in one field were both affecting and being influenced by other fields. So, for example, the increasing professionalization of nursing created the need for a specific body of knowledge which could be called 'nursing knowledge' and which challenged the medical model, while at the same time the medical model was responding to the challenge nursing posed and was increasingly incorporating psychological and sociological knowledge, while these academic disciplines themselves were changing and applying these changes to problems in health and social care.

The biopsychosocial model

Engel (1977) proposed an alternative approach to the biomedical model, which reflected the emergent complexity and multiplicity of understandings of health and illness through the inclusion of biological *and* psychological *and* social factors into what he has termed 'the biopsychosocial model'. Engel summarized this growing sense of unease with the biomedical model when he stated that 'we are now faced with the necessity and the challenge to broaden the approach to disease to include the psycho-social without sacrificing the enormous advantages of the biomedical approach' (ibid., p.130).

The biopsychosocial approach was accepted in both academic and practical spheres, not least because it was felt that this model provided a comprehensive and holistic understanding of individuals' experiences of health and disease. However, when we begin to look at the way in which this approach has been utilized at both the theoretical and practical levels, it soon becomes apparent that the model has itself been interpreted and applied in a diverse number of ways. Indeed, it can be seen that the way in which the model has been applied has been very much dependent on the academic discipline and professional orientation of those who adopt such a model. This can be illustrated by looking at the diversity of the application of the model in professions whose development partially led to the challenge to biomedicine.

The increasing professionalization of occupations such as nursing, social work and health visiting was part of the growing threat to medicine, and these professions were developing their own models to underpin practice. Once the biopsychosocial model has developed, with the psychological and social aspects appended to the biological understandings, this was then diffused into the development of other professional models.

A range of nursing models has developed (Rogers 1970; Orem 1971; Roy 1976; Roper *et al.* 1980; Johnson 1980), some of which, while varying in the way in which the practical aspects of the profession were represented and practised, can be seen to incorporate the ethos of the biopsychosocial model. Models such as these served to establish a framework for nursing that moved away from the earlier, dominant biomedical model towards a much broader understanding that endorsed a multi-level account of health and illness. However, claims of 'holism' made by such models are seriously challenged by criticisms that question the over-importance attributed to biological explanations in many of the models (Aggleton and Chalmers 1986).

While nursing adopted the biopsychosocial model, other professions such as social work, more distanced from medicine, were less committed to it. Following the Seebohm Committee Report (1968), an increasingly formal structure was created around social work, but there was a sense in which the need for a coherent and distinctive body of knowledge was still to be addressed. This lack of unity was reflected in a certain degree of ambivalence around the notion of 'theory', with a subsequent tension between those writers who argued that social work lacked 'theory' and those who maintained that the ideologies and practices of social work were essentially manifestations of a tacit theory-base. That is, while social work may not have carried an explicit theoretical framework underpinning practice, this did not preclude the existence, and influence, of implicit assumptions underlying that practice. Indeed, we can see this latter position being expressed in work that aimed to explore the relationship between such implicit knowledge and the practical skills and theories of social work (Curnock and Hardiker 1979). One facet of this implicit knowledge can be seen in social work's emphasis on values such as self-determination and respect for the person. Indeed, in exploring the relationship between assumptive knowledge and practice, values such as these can be seen to place social work into a framework that is not only informed by the social scientific disciplines of psychology and sociology, but that also reflects the moral ideals extant within any given culture at any given time (Hardiker and Barker 1981). Thus, Hardiker and Barker argue that 'it is because social work models of man [*sic*] are not reducible to social science man that they must rely on more holistic and eclectic perspectives which the word "person" describes rather aptly' (ibid., p.87), and, in so doing, move social work into a moral and cultural domain that demands a more appropriate explanation of related theory and practice. The professions which operate in health and social care therefore differ in their orientation and organization which influences the way in which the biopsychosocial model may be utilized. This also suggests that professionals may subscribe to different meanings associated with the components of the model. That the professionals who draw upon the model use it in different ways is not surprising given that the academic use of the model is demonstrative of the uncertainty of its integration.

The meanings of the model

The central issue that arises from the application of the biopsychosocial model is that concerning potential differences in meaning. How is it interpreted by those who adopt it? One way in which we can explore questions such as these is by focusing on the way in which the concept of a 'biopsychosocial model' is described and utilized within the context of texts in the field of health psychology.

While purporting to adopt an integrated biopsychosocial approach, writers tend to juxtapose knowledge from the three disciplines of biology, sociology and psychology onto the main disciplinary orientation of their own work. Sarafino (1990) states an intention to adopt the biopsychosocial model as the fundamental explanatory theme of his *Health Psychology* textbook. While he goes on to argue that the components of the biopsychosocial model 'interrelate in a dynamic and continuous fashion, consistent with the concept of *system*' (ibid., p.vii), there is little further development of this key conceptualization.

Indeed, neither the notion of different levels of explanation which necessarily follows from this conceptualization, nor the need for reconciliation of these different levels, is acknowledged or addressed by the author. In so doing, the biopsychosocial model is presented as a *multiple*, rather than *integrated*, explanatory framework in which biological, social and psychological factors co-exist in a seemingly fragmented way. And, as it is generally accepted that any 'theory' should be integrative, predictive and capable of organizing knowledge coherently, then it could be argued that the biopsychosocial approach, as described and applied by Sarafino, does not fulfil these requirements. Thus, while the text presents the biopsychosocial model as a theoretical framework, on examination we can see that the model merely reflects the simultaneous juxtaposition of a range of explanatory perspectives and *not* the integrated theoretical model that its status implies.

We can see a somewhat different conceptualization of the model in the work of Sheridan and Radmacher (1992), who attempt to address the issue of levels of explanation and their integration through a location of the biopsychosocial approach within the broader framework of general systems theory. The implication here would be that the biological, social and psychological perspectives that are a part of the model exist complementarily, each one affecting and being affected by change and variation in another.

How, then, does Sheridan and Radmacher's understanding of the biopsychosocial approach stand alongside that of Sarafino? There is a sense in which both conceptualizations are saying the same thing – that is, that understandings of health and illness must be conceptualized in terms of biological, social and psychological factors. However, when it comes to addressing the issue of how these factors interrelate, the contrast between the two approaches is clear. Sheridan and Radmacher attempt to explain this through the adoption of a systemic analysis, whereas Sarafino fails to address the issue at all. Thus, we have a model which, although superficially promising in its comprehensive consideration of influential factors in understanding health and illness, is seriously theoretically flawed in its failure to provide any plausible explanation of the interrelationship between these factors – that is, in how the components of the model 'fit together'. This is very different from the biomedical model of health and disease which has built an apparently cohesive body of knowledge from the scientific disciplines which underpin medical practice.

The hegemony of knowledge: the biomedical model

The dominant representation of 'medicine' is frequently that of a singular entity, bounded within a larger framework of 'scientific knowledge' and sharing a common understanding of both 'the body' and the therapeutic techniques available to support and maintain the health of that body. However, this singular view of medicine can be seen to be the culmination of a long-term sociohistorical process characterized by – and given impetus by – tensions existing at the levels of both practical application and philosophical abstraction (Lawrence 1994). For example, if we look back to the Middle Ages, we see a divide between the surgeon and the physician, not only in the professional kudos attributed to one at the expense of the other, but at the more fundamental level where surgical procedures were seen as being the province of those of a lower socioeconomic status than 'medical men'.

The significance of this basic tension can be seen in its consequences for understanding health and illness. The surgical world was one of pathological anatomical structures being excised in order to understand the relationship between physical symptoms and disease processes. For the physician, however, an alternative emphasis involving observation of the patient's external clinical signs and symptoms was held to be the key to understanding health and illness. Although it is accepted that tensions may remain between these two types of practitioner even today, the contemporary situation is such that both occupations are subsumed under the umbrella profession of medicine. Yet the idea of attempting to bring these two specialities closer together (and thereby eliminating existing tensions) was dismissed as a utopian dream during the Middle Ages (Gelfand 1980).

During the sixteenth century, knowledge of healing came to be founded upon a classical education that reflected the re-emerging importance of classical scholars such as Hippocrates and Galen. Alongside the reconstruction of classical texts on anatomy, physiology and botany, which was ongoing at that time (Wear *et al.* 1985), was a recognition not only of the *relevance* of philosophical theory in this area, but indeed the *importance* of such theories in developing and understanding the practice of medicine. These philosophical aspects have largely lost their significance: 'We have departed a long way from this ideal. Over the years there has been a trend towards skill and away from wisdom, towards training and away from education' (Charlton 1993: 476). Charlton argued that the focus on science which underpins medical training has led to a situation in which doctors have a single mode of thought, the 'medical morality', and he suggested that while medical morality is valuable, it limits the doctor in his or her ability to practise humanely.

While the broad wisdom possessed by the educated doctors of the sixteenth century may therefore be perceived as a strength, the humoral theories drawn from classical knowledge which underpinned medicine had difficulties in accommodating specific conditions such as plague and the 'new' disease of syphilis. Consequently, although humoral explanations may have dominated this period, there was a sense in which this provided only a limited understanding of many medical conditions and, as a result, we see that a reliance on occult systems, with their associated religious and/or magical interventions, was still very much in evidence (Fissell 1991). By the seventeenth century, however, medicine began to challenge religious ideas with intellectual and ethical issues and conditions once regarded as occult were increasingly seen as a medical problem. Medical theories became mechanical, but there was a continued inability to account for certain phenomena, which meant that medicine did not achieve total dominance. Medicine's hegemony of knowledge in health was firmly established with the ascension of science over religion towards the mid- to late eighteenth century. Foucault (1963/73) argued that this medical 'gaze' had become so powerful by this time that most, if not all, alternative conceptualizations of health and illness were undermined and/or discredited by its near ubiquitous acceptance in Western society. Developments in science continued to influence medicine until, towards the end of the nineteenth century, we see one further major change that served to affirm the position of medical knowledge.

The field of laboratory science and the establishment of 'germ theory' began to exert an influence on the understanding and treatment of disease, specifically the control of diseases of epidemic scale. The development of germ theory could also be incorporated into other biological theories such as cell theory and evolution to provide an integrated body of complementary knowledge. The capability of laboratory sciences in general, and the cell theories in particular, provided a context within which disease could be understood, and led King (1982: 297) to conclude that 'the great progress in bacteriology probably did more to underscore the importance of science in medicine than did any other single advance'. Scientific medicine had arrived. Medical schools increasingly drew on this new and exciting scientific representation of disease, with the result that a unitary group of medical practitioners began to form who were grounded in a similar scientific base and trained with similar professional skills. Hence we see the beginnings of a process of formalization of the biomedical model, a process which reached its peak in the mid-twentieth century.

Within the biomedical approach, healthy people become manifestations of healthy cellular activity; ill people become manifestations of dysfunctional cellular (i.e. bacteriological) activity. The patient becomes a 'problem' to be solved, and the solution to that problem lies in adopting a scientific, mechanistic approach that precludes any consideration of social, psychological or behavioural influences.

The growing confidence in this model of health and illness therefore was not without its shadow side. The identification of the medical profession with a scientific understanding of health and disease can be seen to have both opened up *and* constrained the way in which illness was conceptualized. For example, one consequence of this alliance between medicine and science was to prevent the practitioner from expressing a commitment to 'people' (McCormick 1979). As medicine and the biomedical model became established as the dominant mode of thought in health and disease, so a challenge to this perspective began to emerge.

The challenge to medical hegemony

Many academic developments have challenged the dominance of the biomedical model. Parsons (1951) conceptualized 'health' as being a necessary and functional requirement of any social system. This particular understanding of health is based on the interrelatedness of individuals and the culture in which they live. Healthy people both sustain and are sustained by a healthy social system, and as such there is a need to take into account cultural, structural and interactional variables affecting health and illness, rather than focusing exclusively on individual factors as is implied by the biomedical model. However, Parsons' model was predicated on a positivist, biomedical model, with problems to be explored being considered relevant by the providers of medical care. Consequently, Parsons' work may be considered to perpetuate the hegemony, although it did begin to draw attention to non-medical factors affecting issues in health and illness.

The early dis-ease with the biomedical model found its strength in the early to mid-1970s, when the model's limitations began to be appreciated and explored more fully (Research Unit in Health and Behavioural Change 1989). Academic discourse began to focus upon, and challenge, the biomedical model's inherent assumption of its own 'objectivity' in particular, and the existence of 'objective knowledge' in general, thereby calling into question the fundamental assumptions on which the biomedical model was based. This led to a critique focused on the implications of such assumptions in construing medically defined appropriate behaviours. That is, if we 'know' what causes illness X, then we 'know' what the appropriate action is to be taken by both patient and practitioner. We also 'know' what is inappropriate action, and thus we begin to see the constraining quality of the model. Can we 'know'? If we answer in the affirmative, then *whose* knowledge informs what is 'known'? Questions such as these served to move the debate towards an exploration of the value-laden nature of the model. For example, Zola (1977) argued that there are three fundamental values underlying 'medical science': activism, worldliness and instrumentalism. Respectively, these values can be seen to be reflected in medicine's powerful need to *act on* the environment rather than *to adjust to* that environment. Hence we find a situation where the aim of medical treatment is to cure, with little if any attempt being made to facilitate patients in managing their conditions within the context of everyday life. Similarly, there is an explicit preference for secular explanation and response to illness, with little acknowledgement of the role played by religious/spiritual aspects of patients' experiences. Finally, Zola argues that medical science is based on an instrumentalism which requires that the practitioner must be seen to be doing something, anything, if her or his credibility and position is to be maintained.

Thus we can see that medicine is not value-free, either at the theoretical level around issues of power in the very definitions of health and illness, or at the practical level of medical practice and the assumptions which underlie and direct such practice. The objective, scientific interpretations ascribed to the biomedical model were rapidly being challenged in such a way as to highlight its lack of flexibility and consequent limitations as an explanatory framework within which health and illness could be understood in an holistic way.

However, developments such as these do not occur in isolation; change occurs within a broader sociocultural context, which is itself subject to a process of constant negotiation and reconstruction. For example, while the limitations of the biomedical model of health and illness were being highlighted in this way, similar debates were taking place in a range of disciplines (e.g. psychology and sociology) with the development of modes of analysis such as symbolic interactionism and social constructionism, in which the importance of considering 'the person in context' was highlighted.

The developments in discourses within the social sciences especially found application in fields such as health and social care. One result of these developing discourses was the suggestion that definitions of health and illness should not be treated as objectively observed and defined 'givens', but as dynamic, socially constructed phenomena created, recreated and negotiated through everyday interaction (Dingwall 1976). Indeed, there is a sense in which Dingwall's observations reflect a development of earlier work on the subjective meaning of social action. For example, Schutz (1972) argued for the dynamic nature of individuals' subjective interpretation of experience and, in so doing, highlighted the person as a conscious and reflective actor attempting to make sense of bodily changes within a framework of his or her own lay knowledge of health and illness. Also within the 1970s a literature began to develop which explored the relationship between the physical body and the social body. So for example, Douglas (1970) developed an analysis of how the physical body may provide a foundation for classificatory systems and how the social world may reflect the perception of the physical body. Such work provided a basis for the development in the sociology of the body in the 1980s (Turner 1984).

These changes also suggested that people could be *studied* in an holistic way, and within academic discourse an associated development in research methodology occurred with the growth of qualitative research strategies. Qualitative techniques provided a greater potential for acknowledging power dynamics inherent in research and frequently produced a different relationship between researcher and subject, which was especially given prominence in feminist writing (Webb 1984). Much feminist writing oriented around a critique of biomedicine as a form of social control (Ehrenreich and English 1973). This feminist critique of the medicalization of women's experience has developed into a discourse which provides an alternative view of health.

Thus, we begin to see a move away from the position of biomedicine as *the* way in which health and illness could be understood, towards the position in which the potential multiplicity of models of health and illness is both recognized and accepted. In so doing, this form of challenge served to disclose the exclusive and singular quality of the biomedical model itself. This challenge to existing positivist conceptions of human behaviour proposed the seemingly simplistic, though apparently radical, notion that human beings can and should be regarded in an holistic way.

The aforementioned academic developments were mirrored in practice with the development of health care professions, and their need to establish research bases and models to underpin practice. It is to an examination of two professions, nursing and social work, that we turn next.

The biopsychosocial model in nursing and social work

During the 1960s, it was increasingly recognized that nursing research needed to intensify:

In most professions we take for granted the existence of research . . .
The amount of research carried out by the profession is small; there has
been little formal assistance with this. Nurses have always assisted their
medical colleagues to collect data, yet seldom have they been fully
involved. They have a very definitive contribution to make to collaborative research.

(Stephenson 1964: 267)

This recognition originated in the increasing professionalization of nursing.
The concept of the professional nurse as advocated by Florence Nightingale
was very much defined by its association with medicine as the focus for the
identification and treatment of disease (Garmanikow 1978). During the
early part of the twentieth century, nursing gradually outgrew its depend-
ence on medicine to develop and formalize its own structures of professionalism, including the introduction of well-defined entry, examination and
registration requirements for those training and practising within the field.
From the 1950s onwards, we begin to see the evolution of conceptual
frameworks within which nursing theory and practice can operate. Nursing
in this period 'felt compelled to eschew all things medical, particularly the
disease orientation and the medical model as the source of nursing concepts'
(Kikuchi and Simmons 1992: 1).

Many models were developed to underpin nursing practice (Rogers 1970;
Orem 1971; Roy 1976; Johnson 1980; Roper et al. 1980). These models
varied in the way they drew on practical task aspects of nursing, and in the
extent to which they incorporated the biopsychosocial model, either implicitly or explicitly. For example, the Activities of Daily Living (ADL)
model (Roper et al. 1980) incorporated an explicit recognition of the interrelationships between activities that were considered to be biological. Aggleton and Chalmers (1986) considered that this model was too biologically
oriented, through its connection to physiological systems (Lister 1987).
Conversely, in Roy's model of adaptation, the person was perceived as 'a
biosocial being' (Roy 1976: 11), and the adaptive process was considered at
the physiological, individual and social levels. The model was also conceptualized in terms of a system, so that a change in one mode caused change in
other modes. Orem's (1971) model of self-care was also built upon holistic
ideas, with the physical, psychological and social aspects of health being
seen as integral within the individual. Orem's model also incorporated aspects considering issues outside of traditional orthodox medicine such as
health promotion. Some models, such as Rogers' (1970), tried to go beyond
the biopsychosocial parameters and included fields such as religion and
philosophy. In her model of unitary man, Rogers considered that the attempt to arrive at holism through the integration of biology, psychology and
sociology, or through the use of systems theory, fails to consider people as
wholes because the integrity and characteristics of man [sic] 'are more than

and different from the sum of his parts' (Rogers 1970: 47). Thus, some models established a framework for nursing that moved away from the medical model, taking into consideration the social sciences.

Despite nursing developing a research base, and increasingly incorporating philosophical inquiry into research (Kikuchi and Simmons 1992), there is still an imbalance in nurses' contribution to health research: 'The lack of involvement by nurses and midwives in multidisciplinary research and the problems in developing appropriate research . . . are related to traditional structures of power and status' (World Health Organization 1994: 14). This indicates that while nursing is developing professionally, it remains subject to medicine.

Like nursing, the social work profession was developing professionally and trying to establish practice models, but the research base was haphazard (Meyer 1976). Unlike nursing, social work origins are more distant from medicine, and by looking at early understandings of 'social work' it can be considered that the discipline is rooted within a moral discourse, reflecting as it does the moral climate of society in the mid- to late nineteenth century (Abbott and Wallace 1990). Early moral discourse eventually gave way to a 'professional' understanding of social work and of social workers, however the profession needed to find a theory to underpin practice.

Theories of practice within social work began to draw heavily upon the social sciences. But Hardiker and Barker recognized that utilizing any disciplinary knowledge created difficulties in achieving a unified theory:

> Differences within and between academic disciplines produce contrasting models of man [*sic*] . . .
>
> (Hardiker and Barker 1981: 4)

They went on to suggest that knowledge can be used as a system. Similarly, social work authors (Janchill 1969; Hartman 1970; Stein 1974) began to use systems theory as a route to explore the nature of an holistic perspective on health and illness, although the latter lacked a biological element.

The development of social work challenged the medical model in spheres initially occupied by doctors. So, for example, child abuse was initially rediscovered within the medical field, but rapidly became recognized as a problem requiring multi-agency input. Social workers, with their psychodynamic understandings, family and client orientation, became the lead agency workers.

While these professional developments were occurring, medicine was becoming increasingly ineffective in curing chronic diseases. The biomedical model of disease had been perceived as being effective in understanding and eliminating infectious diseases, a major cause of death, although this was contested by McKeown (1976), who suggested that the major decline in infectious diseases had occurred due to improved public hygiene, nutrition and housing. 'Killers' became chronic conditions with multiple causes relating to biological, social and psychological aspects. For example, heart disease is associated with factors such as smoking, lack of exercise, stress and obesity. Medicine, drawing upon biological models, may be able to understand the disease process, but to have any influence on reducing mortality rate, recourse to psychological and social knowledge is necessary.

The appearance of 'new' diseases, such as acquired immune deficiency syndrome (AIDS) and human immunodeficiency virus (HIV), also revealed medicine's inadequacies. Despite the increase in medical knowledge the incidence of HIV continues to grow (Hersh and Peterson 1988). Without a biological solution to AIDS in the immediate future, the strategy for AIDS control is one of primary prevention through health education and health promotion (Phillips 1988).

The biopsychosocial model in health promotion

There is a sense in which the foundations of health promotion are located in a sweeping generalization from the 'medical' to the 'social'. By this we mean that early approaches in this field involved taking ideas of health traditionally associated with medicine and traditionally attributed to the individual, such as the concept of 'hygiene', and then extending these ideas to the social phenomenon of 'a population'. Thus, 'hygiene' is no longer merely an individual issue, but a social issue whereby the causes and consequences of health and illness are construed in terms analogous to the 'disease', 'process' and 'prevention' issues of individual health; these issues are now seen as being located in both the individual's immediate and extended social world. Hence, the health of the individual can no longer be separated from the 'healthiness' of that social world.

Indeed, Lalonde (1974) argued that structural and behavioural changes in society were essential to any significant improvement in a society's level of health. This argument implies a move away from the biomedical focus on disease and illness, towards an understanding of health and health promotion that lies outside of the dominant domain of medical expertise. Thus, we see within the field of health promotion a highlighting of both individual and structural elements, inasmuch as health promotional strategies are reflective of multiple levels of understanding and intervention. This multiplicity can include psychological theory (as it applies to attitude change, for example), an emphasis on behavioural skills (as they apply to health) and an awareness of the need for environmental changes in promoting health in society.

However, this is not to say that health promotion draws only on the social and behavioural sciences; biological aspects, such as epidemiology, can be seen to retain their importance within the field. Indeed, health promotion and health education are now readily accepted as multidisciplinary arenas, within which a wide range of agencies can and do work together:

> . . . the importance of national and local agencies such as the Royal College of Physicians, the BMA and the health education agencies, together with health and local authorities and FHSAs, in taking a lead in the promotion of health has been clearly illustrated in the case of cigarette smoking, and in more recent initiatives to prevent the spread of HIV/AIDS.
>
> (Jacobson *et al.* 1991: 15)

Recent years have seen the formalization of a multidisciplinary approach in the development of a range of models of health promotion (Ewels and Simnett 1985; Tannahill 1985; Caplan and Holland 1990). Health promotion literature also raises the issue of lay explanations of health and illness, and there is a sense in which the development of health promotion as a subject area has both drawn on and contributes towards such explanations. The importance of lay understandings of health and illness is reflected in Jacobson and co-workers' comment that 'the need to promote a willing partnership between users and professionals in the promotion of health is enshrined in the NHS and Community Care Act' (Jacobson *et al.* 1991: 15). Thus, if health promotion strategies are to be effective, the cooperation of those receiving such strategies is essential and, in turn, if those receivers are to cooperate, then health promotion 'knowledge' must be made accessible and meaningful. In so doing, health promotion and health education serve to challenge practitioners to share their knowledge, to cross that expert/lay boundary which can often be so firmly entrenched in the notion of 'professionalism'. Arguably, then, it is in health promotion that we see a clear illustration of how the limitations of a medicalized, scientific model of health and illness can and must be addressed if the work of practitioners in this area is to be taken on board by those to whom such work is directed.

Alternative 'caring' and the biopsychosocial model

So far, we have looked at developments located within the general domain of disciplines and professions. However, when we begin to look at the more specific areas within those disciplines and professions, we can see a similar progression from a dominance ascribed to biomedically informed models of health and illness to the contemporary situation whereby a multiplicity of understandings are extant within the culture at any given time. A clear example of this can be seen in the area of palliative care, in which we can see concerns with the limitations of the biomedical model being expressed and acted upon formally in the move towards an holistic model of care and the setting up of institutions within which such care could be practised. As Dame

Cicely Saunders (1977: 164) comments, 'I am not only concerned with what is yours (your diagnosis, your response to treatment and so on) but with you as a person (however despairing you are, however unattractive)'.

This simple statement has since come to represent the fundamental ethos of the hospice 'philosophy of care'. The Hospice Movement can be traced back to the mid-nineteenth century founded by Mary Aikenhead and the Irish Sisters of Charity, who perceived the need of a nursing home where a peaceful environment could be created and which, despite being smaller in size, was able to offer the same level of nursing care as could be found within the more formal, and less peaceful, hospital situation.

These developments can be seen to come to fruition in the 1950s with the establishment of the Marie Curie Foundation. Thus, we see the formalization of the hospice ethos; those who are dying can now be said to receive an holistic response whether at home or, as may become necessary, in the institutional context of in-patient care. This holistic response has been summarized by Biswas (1993) in the following way:

- a recognition that dying is not a symptom but a process, *and that people need more than just physical care*;
- a recognition of *the role of family and friends* and the impact on them of the patient's process of dying and subsequent death;
- a recognition of *the contributions needed from a range of disciplines* in order that all needs are to be met – emotional, spiritual and social in addition to the physical needs of the dying person;
- a recognition that *death does not need to be seen as a negative experience*, but that it can be a positive and enriching experience.

Thus, we can see a very similar story taking place within the specific area of palliative care that we have already seen in the broader fields of nursing and social work. The dominance of the biomedical model of care has been challenged significantly by the call for a more holistic approach, with the consequence that the plausibility of this medical perspective alone in explaining and understanding health, illness, death and dying has become increasingly difficult to sustain.

The growth in interest in and, to some extent, the credibility of complementary medicine can be seen to epitomize this increasing unease around the explanatory power of biomedicine and its associated models of health and illness. Indeed, the change in terminology from 'alternative' to 'complementary' almost parallels the way in which the biopsychosocial model has evolved from being an alternative model of health to being a model which not only complements biomedical approaches but, in fact, incorporates such approaches. Complementary medicine can be seen to have followed a similar path, whereby its position *outside* of the traditional 'camp' of medical practice has developed in recent years to one in which a wide range of complementary therapies can be made available *within* that traditional camp. Hence, health practice can be seen to have incorporated 'holistic' therapies in much the same way as health theory has begun to acknowledge and adopt the more holistic biopsychosocial approach.

When we begin to look at the historical context within which complementary therapy developed, it is interesting to note that the sociocultural climate of the time was, arguably, the least conducive to such a development. As Saks (1992: 8) comments: 'At the beginning of the 1960's [the] medical hegemony was rather more complete and a negative view tended to be reflexively taken of alternative practitioners by both the public and medical establishment alike'.

However, despite this, the same period saw a growth of interest in alternative lifestyles, with the influence of Eastern cultures being particularly apparent. The increasing awareness of non-traditional ways of 'being' served to create a climate in which the relationship between physical and psychological selves became the focus for exploration and understanding. It soon became clear that traditional representations of health and associated practices were inappropriate to this holistic emphasis, and thus we see a growing number of individuals searching for therapies which, and practitioners who, were consistent with such an holistic approach.

By the early 1980s, complementary medicine was seen both as an expanding field in terms of its available body of knowledge (Fulder and Monro 1981) and as a growth industry, inasmuch as more and more people were moving into its associated therapies and practices. Complementary practice could no longer be marginalized or dismissed as a passing whim. Conventional medicine responded defensively to these developments. The proportion of people consulting practitioners in this area had reached the point where the earlier sweeping criticisms of complementary practice were replaced by a more specific attack on the efficacy of its associated therapies. Thus, the British Medical Association (BMA 1986: 75) argued that 'new and unconventional techniques should be evaluated with the same methods that have been applied to therapeutic methods now known, through the results of careful evaluation, to be effective'.

While this might be seen as a step forwards in an acceptance of complementary approaches by conventional medicine, there is a sense in which such a statement reflects the entire thesis of both this chapter and this book – that is, the assumption of an 'objectivity' which exists within a phenomenon and which is therefore open to 'careful evaluation'. The present authors' argument is concisely summed up in complementary medicine's response to this assumption – that is, that 'science is not an objective reality, it is constructed as a social entity by persons' (British Holistic Medical Association 1986: 69). It is fascinating to note the parallels between this statement, located as it is in the 'conventional versus complementary' medicine debate, and the statement expressed within the context of social constructionist movements within academic discourse. For example Gergen

(1985: 267) stated that 'the terms in which the world is understood are social artefacts products of historically situated interchanges among people'. Here we see a more global representation of the BHMA statement; it is not merely 'science' that defies the assumption of objectivity, but, according to Gergen, 'the world' in its entirety must be understood in a similar way if we are to approach an understanding of human action in any authentic way.

Thus, we can see that complementary medicine, while developing within the specific context of dissatisfaction with conventional medicine, is reflective of a far broader conflict of ethos existing between biomedical and holistic approaches.

Conclusion

The major mode of understanding in health and disease has recently shifted from a situation in which there was a dominant biomedical explanation, to a position in which different forms of knowledge are accepted and regarded as necessary to fully understand health and illness.

The biopsychosocial model has evolved as one expression of the attempt to bring together these diverse understandings of health and illness. The model has developed in the context of a general questioning of the ability of biomedicine to account for and cure disease. This included: the growth of academic critiques that doubted the existence of objective, value-free knowledge; the challenge from other professions as they underwent a process of professionalization; general social change reflected in such movements as the development of alternative forms of caring in relation to death and dying; and growing acceptance of complementary therapies which attempted an 'holistic' response to those with biological needs. The relationship between the development of the biopsychosocial model, academic disciplines, the professions, and social change was dynamic, with changes in each of these areas both adapting to and affecting the others. This process is therefore difficult to describe in linear terms.

Prior to these changes medicine, as a unitary science-based profession, enjoyed an uncontested high status. The development of the biopsychosocial model by 'adding on' the psychological and the social to biological understandings has helped to preserve biomedicine and has prevented it from being sacrificed on the altar of social science. Medicine therefore can be seen to have accepted some 'scientific' social and psychological knowledge while remaining largely entrenched within a biological framework. Nursing has also maintained a strong allegiance to biology, but has drawn extensively on psychology and sociology in an effort to develop and substantiate a theoretical aspect to nursing care which distinguished nursing from medicine. Social work has been less constrained by a biological 'history' and so has sought to develop knowledge based largely upon the social sciences and moral ideas. The biopsychosocial model is therefore a social product which is utilized in different ways depending upon the professional orientation. How interactions between the components of this model operate is rarely addressed; rather the balance of orientation towards one explanatory perspective is generally preferred by a whole profession. However in everyday practice professionals may use whatever perspective appears to 'work' with a situation, in a pragmatic fashion.

The biopsychosocial model developed in response to a rising critique of the limitations of the biomedical model, but little attention was paid to how the former could be implemented in practice. Practitioners have been left to find their own strategies to manage the tensions between the different forms of knowledge inherent in the model. For workers in the real world, the biopsychosocial model raises as many difficulties as it resolves. This is reflected in the practitioners' narratives of their everyday experience as reported in the chapters in Part 1.

While the biopsychosocial model more accurately portrays the experience of clients, it has limitations in relation to holistic practice and in turn raises the question 'what is holism?' Is it possible for any model to incorporate holism or is holism more useful as a general framework within which biopsychosocial care may be enacted?

The relationship between the biopsychosocial model and everyday practice in health and social care is complex, and this relationship forms the basis of the exploration of the biopsychosocial model and the integration of perspectives on health in the following chapters.

Part 1

Professional perspectives and practice

Introduction

This part of the book concerns the application of the biopsychosocial model within professional practice. In Chapter 2, Pauline Pearson draws upon her professional experience of health visiting to construct a description of the way in which health visitors attempt to reconcile different explanations of health behaviour within their practice.

Pauline shows how the different aspects of the biopsychosocial model may be utilized to explain the health behaviours of clients. Looking back on practice situations, she reveals a feeling of 'loose ends' with respect to certain issues, such as the political and economic influences on health. She goes on to consider health visiting in relation to three specific practice areas: health promotion, child health and the care of the elderly. Taking up the shortcomings of the biopsychosocial model to address political and wider social concerns, Pauline sets out a potential role for the health visitor in the field of health promotion, and illustrates how health visiting changes to meet client need. With respect to the key area of child health, she demonstrates how health visitors have a critical role in the identification of children with special needs. In considering work with the elderly, she contrasts the biomedical approach to that of a biopsychosocial model. She shows how a consideration of the needs of the elderly, which includes psychological and social dimensions, is superior to that imposed on a health visiting role constrained by a biomedical model. Pauline suggests that the integration of the biopsychosocial explanations do not occur at a theoretical level, but that the different explanations 'work' when used pragmatically in practice. Further integration may be facilitated by the health visitors themselves, as they hold a unique position which bridges the health and social professions.

In Chapter 3, John Fulton considers the influence of the biopsychosocial model on nursing theory and practice by drawing on substantive theory inducted through his own research. While being well accepted in academic and educational nursing environments, the biopsychosocial model is not uniformly applied in practice. Psychosocial caring is subjugated to physical caring. John explores whether the tension between theory and practice, or between the ideal and reality of caring, is due to a lack of commitment to the biopsychosocial model on the part of nurses. Alternatively, he asks, are there other reasons for the deficit in practice?

In his chapter, John sets out evidence that nurses recognize the ideal of the biopsychosocial model of caring. Simultaneously, they are aware of the emotional demands of caring that go beyond the 'physical'. According to John, the recognition of the gap between 'ideal and real' leads nurses to construct accounts for why the deficits in caring occur. Sometimes resource shortages are invoked; however, the main justification is couched in a self-serving assertion of the caring nature of their own nursing activity.

Through considering professional differences within multidisciplinary teams in Chapter 4, Chris Stevenson and Phil Barker assert that a wealth of explanations for 'invisible' mental health problems are possible. They range from the social structural to the individual pathological, with interpersonal theories also included. The explanations derive from the attitudes and value systems of various disciplines that cross paths with so-called 'sufferers'. The diversity of explanations is now being seriously reviewed by practitioners who are 'thrown together' by multidisciplinary team working, which has increased with legislation in the 1980s and 1990s, leading to the closure of large psychiatric hospitals. This is especially the case in community care settings, where community psychiatric nurses (CPNs), social workers, psychologists, psychiatrists and occupational therapists are obliged to find ways to practise in unison.

Chris and Phil note that one explanation is not necessarily better than any other. However, there is a strong rationalist, empiricist tradition in Western society that favours materialism over explanations that are less reductionist (e.g. subjective assessments of the world).

The authors propose that disciplines which can claim 'scientific knowledge' are in a powerful position in relation to other disciplines. There is a knowledge/power hierarchy. The hierarchy is visible in some well-rehearsed aspects of caring. When the hierarchy is institutionalized, it may become self-sustaining, as the different disciplines fall into specific roles appropriate to their perceived power position. Chris and Phil share their concern that when specific disciplines are narrowly defined within the team, their creativity in practice is limited, to the cost of multidisciplinary working. When disciplines do create ways to work together, however, it is a fascinating process. Chris and Phil use a social constructionist analysis to unpack the ways in which roles are defined through client–professional and professional–professional interaction.

However, social constructionism may simply 'paper over' the duality of different explanations of the world. Chris and Phil argue that there is value in accepting the problematic nature of knowledge. Alternative paradigms promote a sufficiently sophisticated array of views to respect the complexity of people who have mental health problems.

Neil Cooper and Allison McInnes continue to consider multidisciplinary action in Chapter 5. This chapter is concerned with the theoretical models that have developed in the understanding of child abuse and neglect. Neil and Allison show that models which represent the different components of the biopsychosocial model have been integrated into an eclectic professional model to explain abuse, as the different periods in the 'rediscovery' of child abuse have required different explanatory frameworks. They illustrate that the modern origins of professional intervention in child abuse occurred with the biomedical model. As child abuse management evolved, it became more multidisciplinary in nature, and as different forms of abuse (e.g. sexual and ritual abuse) emerged, the biomedical approach, and its associated explanations, increasingly came to be challenged. The psychological and social aspects of abuse became appended to the biomedical approach to form a body of knowledge that may guide professional intervention. As intervention strategies were developed from a basis in biomedicine, the alternative strategies of management that could be utilized from the developing psychological and social understandings were constrained. Neil and Allison argue that, because professionals have to manage abuse, the different levels of explanation have formed into an amorphous professional model that can be shaped to fit any individual case through professional negotiation. In common with the position Pauline Pearson takes in Chapter 2 regarding theory and practice, Neil and Allison argue that the biopsychosocial model works in practice, but falls short of an integrated model, and as the model operates from a biomedical foundation, the potential for an holistic approach to child abuse cannot be achieved within current frameworks.

2

Health visiting: a profession for all seasons

Pauline Pearson

Introduction

Just as Thomas More is described as 'the man for all seasons' by Robert Bolt, so health visitors can be seen as professionals for all seasons, at least in their adaptability to changing contexts and their eclectic use of theory. This chapter begins by outlining briefly what health visiting is about. It looks at the principles of health visiting and indicates ways in which a variety of theoretical models may be applied in practice. Three high-profile areas of practice are discussed – health promotion and the public health, child health and the care of the elderly. Issues and stresses arising from the application of diverse and sometimes divergent theories are highlighted. The emergence of a unified biopsychosocial model is discussed. Changes and challenges for theory emerging from current developments in community nursing and primary care are set out.

What is health visiting about?

The general public is very unclear about health visitors and their role (Pearson 1988a). Health visitors are registered nurses who have undertaken a further year's course in higher education to enable them to work in the community with a particular brief for promoting health and preventing illness. Much of their time is spent visiting children under five and their families (Clark 1973; Dunnell and Dobbs 1983), but they are also involved with other age groups, particularly elderly people. They are usually employed by community units or Trusts, but often attached to general practitioner (GP) practices. Together with GPs, district nurses, practice nurses and practice managers, they form the core of the so-called 'primary health care team' (Pearson and Jones 1994). All this sounds very straightforward. However, the reality is more complex. Why?

Lack of clarity about our role may be because we are uncertain ourselves (Goodwin 1982), but perhaps also because of the flexibility that has been our greatest strength. Over the past hundred years, health visitors have moved from being local community leaders to sanitary inspectors (Dingwall *et al*. 1988), to specialists in child development and parenting (DHSS 1976), to authorities in health promotion (Macleod Clark 1993). The key to this set of moves lies in the principles of health visiting, first addressed in 1977 by the Council for the Education and Training of Health Visitors and recently revisited by Twinn and Cowley (1992). They are:

- The search for health needs,
- stimulation of the awareness of health needs,
- the influence on policies affecting health, *and*
- the facilitation of health-enhancing activities.

They remain as relevant today as in 1977. In focusing on health rather than disease, the importance of the biopsychosocial model is immediately apparent. Health can be defined biologically, psychologically, socially, or all three. The World Health Organization's (1978) definition of health – 'a state of complete physical, mental and social well-being' – encapsulates this, and is usually seen as the most useful overall definition for health visitors. In order to search for health needs, to influence policies about health or to facilitate health-enhancing activities, health must be a clearly understood concept. Health needs in the community change – and with them, health visiting must change. Perceptions of health need and views on health-enhancing activity also alter, and health visiting must shift to influence and facilitate people. At the same time, the theories underpinning practice metamorphose.

The ideas underpinning health visiting practice are drawn from a wide spectrum of sources. Biological concepts (e.g. in areas relating to immunology) may be found alongside psychological and sociological concepts, such as discussions about the impact of poverty on smoking (Blackburn 1993) or ideas about reinforcement of healthy lifestyles (Pender *et al*. 1990). In Chapter 1, the notion has been put forward that a biopsychosocial model of health has been developed in an attempt to create a coherent entity in professional practice, both in medicine as it acknowledged its own inability to cure certain diseases, and in orbital professions. This is not obvious on a day-to-day level. The theories upon which I have drawn consciously are taken from many areas, and often appear to be incompatible with each other, let alone the perspectives of other professionals. Yet in reflecting upon them and making sense of my practice, it is in the practice itself that they become coherent – joined by their ability, together, to make sense of what I do.

Health promotion and the public health

Facilitating people in health-enhancing activities has always been at the heart of health visiting practice. Since the early 1970s, this approach has been labelled 'health promotion', enabling people to achieve their full potential for health by giving them greater control over activities and policies affecting health. Ashton and Seymour (1988) outline the way in which the ideas of Illich (1975) on the iatrogenic nature of modern medicine, together with increasing demographic and economic pressures, led to a reappraisal of the health care priorities of the early 1970s and the development of the 'new' public health. In the latter, individual and environmental approaches are combined, with a clear recognition that the environment is social and psychological as well as physical. Preventive measures are used alongside steps to bring about environmental change and together with appropriate levels of therapeutic intervention. Health promotion is central to putting the new public health into practice. Health visitors have been in the vanguard of this.

Since the late 1970s, health visitors have been involved in community development for health. Though the earliest health visitors were community-based, looking at the health needs of particular localities, with the move towards general practice attachment after the 1974 Health Service reorganization, much of the wider community dimension of health visiting seemed to be lost. Yet, day by day, the community context formed a subtext to contacts with individuals and families. It was in projects set up by a few innovative people that health visitors began to reclaim their skills in this area, and consider what health promotion in the community really meant.

My own experience in the early 1980s in the Riverside Child Health Project, established by a forward-thinking paediatrician, Mike Downham, was probably fairly typical (Pearson 1988b). I had been qualified as a health visitor for just over a year when I moved to the project, where I joined a team of doctors, a social worker, a community worker and two secretaries. Our aim was to promote child health in an identifiably disadvantaged area of Newcastle. Coming from a variety of professional perspectives, we looked at a number of approaches to this.

I worked with a small caseload of families, undertaking routine visits and dealing with many problems associated with poverty and deprivation. The father of a child visited routinely for developmental surveillance might be unemployed, struggling to find a new and valid role in society. On an individual level, his relationship to the processes of society (e.g. employment, division of household labour, etc.) altered. In one such family I visited, a man's wife took up paid part-time work, with the result that her husband became responsible for housework and child care. After a few months, the psychological impact of this shift in traditional gender roles became unacceptable to both of them, and she gave up work. Later on, the husband took up a new and unsuccessful 'career' as a burglar – perhaps the lure of once again being able to provide for his family in the way which society seems to expect, and the opportunity of theft came together to engineer his 'deviant' behaviour. He went to prison, and his wife was left to cope with the psychological and social stresses of single parenthood. A biological approach to assessing the health needs of this family clearly would only provide a limited and superficial understanding. At no time did they suffer from organic illness. The children manifested some minor behavioural changes, but continued to develop well within normal limits. They seemed to be loved and cared for. However, the impact of the shift in roles on both of the parents was significant. Support in the several changes which followed the initial job loss required me to understand the psychological impact of life transitions (Felner *et al.* 1980) and to integrate my understanding of the sociological literature on gender and work (Open University U205 course team). While each individual needed support in managing his or her own stresses, for which I could draw on psychological understandings, the family as a whole needed to be looked at, in terms of its function, for which I drew upon sociological theories.

Situated outside the normal primary health care team structure, I debated my management of 'my' families with the social worker in the team. This seemed to be a more appropriate mechanism for routine reflection than discussion with the doctors in the team. Perhaps this was because my perspectives on health were more grounded in social and psychological theories than in medical models. Social workers, even more than health visitors, have a strong belief in the value of peer supervision (Payne and Scott 1990), and my colleague was used to working in this way.

As well as providing enhanced medical and nursing care, another of our objectives was 'to encourage parents and the wider community to assume a greater share of responsibility for their children's health'. Later in the project we spent time explaining that this objective was about empowerment, not about blame. I began to visit local groups and to discuss health issues with them. At first I went into the groups with my own health promotion agendas. I wanted to look at health in pregnancy, and to do work on weaning. The groups were less interested in these topics: they wanted me to talk about first-aid, their own perceived health problems (e.g. successful dieting) and how to cope with sleep disturbance or tantrums. As time went on, they wanted to talk about their experiences of dealing with authority figures (e.g. health professionals, DSS offices, housing officials) and to express their concerns about their community (e.g. children who may be being abused, dogs roaming the streets, glue sniffers, lack of play-space, break-ins). Reflecting on those discussions now, more than ten years later, I think that while over time I became more accepted within the group, my role changed from being a professional 'expert' to being a relatively powerless participant in struggling with the dilemmas of daily life. In the areas (essentially in health care) where the project had power we addressed change, but we did little to alter the attitudes of DSS officials, or to deal with glue sniffing and stray dogs.

Orr (1985) outlines three models of community participation: *marginal participation*, in which professionals remain the 'experts', but the community are involved through representation; *community-based initiatives*, in which the role of the professional is to provide people in a community with a clearer understanding of what they can do to improve health; and the *self-help* model, in which the group defines its own terms of reference and professional roles are peripheral.

In my work with groups at Riverside, I moved through each of these models, but with little idea of where I was going. This may have been because despite my affinity for social and psychological models when working at an individual or family level, at a community level I was still bound by a more limited concept of health, more medically defined, than I now hold. I was happy to offer the women in the groups psychological support, and help them to analyse their experiences in a limited social context. I was less able to analyse their experiences at a community level and thus facilitate appropriate responses. Perhaps my understanding of the interrelationships between social policy, politics, economics and health was still in its infancy. Perhaps the management structures of the time did not facilitate me in developing a broader perspective. When I look back, I see many loose ends.
✴ Health visitors working in community development now approach practice differently. In their account of the public health post at Strelley in Nottingham, Boyd *et al.* (1993) set out the way in which they developed a community profile and analysed the key health needs and appropriate levels of strategic and operational response. Organizational theories back up their understanding of social policy and of the social and environmental influences on health. As well as working with individuals and groups on behaviour change in relation to food, for example, they use networking between community groups involved in resource and service provision to enable local people to influence policies affecting health, for example supermarkets' purchasing policy.

Health promotion in primary care teams

Most health visitors, at least outside London, work in 'primary health care teams', attached to general practitioners. The *Health of the Nation* report (DoH 1992) with its emphasis on health promotion, followed by the publication of the new GP Contract (DoH and Welsh Office 1989) and the development of monitoring of the health promotion work of general practice, led to radical shifts in the thinking of many GPs. The development of the purchaser–provider model in health care, greater awareness of the costs of current models of acute care and moves to shift resources into the community have contributed to an analysis that sees the promotion of health and prevention of ill health, together with the effective management of chronic disease, as central to the future of primary care.

The *Health of the Nation* sets out targets to be achieved for the public's health. For example, it requires that teenage pregnancies (under sixteen years of age) be reduced by 50 per cent by the year 2000. Having laid out what it sees as needing to be achieved, the document goes on to make explicit the need for health professionals to work in partnership – 'healthy alliances' – with other agencies. Just as the biological perspective is inadequate to fully explain either health or illness, so health professionals alone cannot hope to achieve the changes required to achieve the *Health of the Nation* targets. For example, many accidents involving children occur on the roads. Ways of reducing these will include partnerships with police in educating children about safe use of roads and partnerships with local authorities and communities to develop traffic-calming measures. Such partnerships require the integration of some diverse notions about health and well-being. However, at the centre of the *Health of the Nation* document is still a very individually oriented biological/psychological idea of health. On the whole it is intervention with individuals and individual changes which are seen as necessary. Partnerships are primarily seen as necessary because health professionals are seen as illness professionals, and it is recognized that influence must be exerted upon well people. The absence of any analysis of the impact of poverty or social class on health demonstrates the reluctance of the government to espouse a more social model of health. Collectively, health visitors have expressed their concern about this omission (*Health Visitors' Journal* 1991).

The 1990 GP Contract stated that GPs and their colleagues should undertake health assessments and clinics to encourage healthy lifestyles in individual patients. The number of practice nurses soared (Ross *et al.* 1994) as GPs employed them to run health promotion clinics. Family Health Service Authorities (FHSAs) employed health promotion facilitators (usually health visitors) to train and encourage practice nurses in undertaking this task. Meanwhile, health visitors were increasingly feeling marginalized.

Concerns about the lack of clear value for money in the mushrooming of health promotion clinics in general practice led to an amended GP Contract in 1993 (NHS Management Executive 1993). From April 1993, three 'bands' were introduced, each representing a level of activity in relation to health promotion. Band 1 involved the collection of basic data about smoking for the adult population of each practice. Band 2 demanded not only the collection of such data but also the minimization of morbidity and mortality in heart disease. Band 3, which it was thought only a handful of practices would attempt to achieve, required the fulfilment of both of the above criteria, together with evidence of active, planned and targeted primary preventive intervention. In reality, most practices opted to try for this. At the same time health visitors saw an opportunity to get involved.

For the health visitor, drawing up a profile of the practice population and identifying areas of health need is almost routine. One health visitor locally drew together the formal and informal information held by the members of her practice to demonstrate areas of health need. Her analysis was buttressed by awareness of ideas about class divisions and family structure, factors preventing disease and influencing health behaviour, and the potential impact of poverty and unemployment. All of these were integrated in the final profile, which included data on pockets of high unemployment, areas with poor housing, areas without accessible leisure facilities, patients with low compliance with immunization programmes, patients who smoked or used to smoke and patients with high blood pressure.

However, in developing a health promotion plan for the practice, each member of the team has different priorities. The midwife's priority (DoH 1993) is the promotion of healthy pregnancy. The district nurse is primarily interested in tertiary prevention, often working with people who already have a chronic disease or disability to prevent complications, and with carers (Buckeldee 1989). The practice nurse may be most interested in promoting women's health (Atkin *et al.* 1993), though many will also be involved in developing effective immunization programmes.

Health visitors could potentially work to promote the health of any part of the practice population. However, their priorities are likely to be shaped by three considerations. First, their own 'routine' work brings them into contact primarily with young families, at a time when they are vulnerable psychologically, socially and physically (Graham and McKee 1980) and potentially open to lifestyle change (Evans 1987). Health promotion activity with young families also offers the opportunity of influencing two generations at once. Second, they will tend to prioritize groups with which other team members are not working and which are high priority for the practice. In this way, they may highlight elderly people not known to the district nurse or GP, or men who are overweight. Third, their own specific skills and interests will be important in their perceptions of priority.

The GP's priorities for health promotion will primarily be those which can be managed opportunistically. He or she is likely to highlight areas where relatively strong scientific evidence exists for the effectiveness of interventions. Charlton *et al.* (1994), a group of doctors including GPs and purchasers, have suggested the use of indicative prevalences to help in deciding upon areas to target. They suggest that health promotion activity should focus on areas that offer best value for money. Thus, coronary artery bypass grafts are very expensive, but because so few are carried out in the average practice, are worthwhile. Brief advice to stop smoking by a GP is effective in around 10 per cent of cases (Fowler 1993) and can be delivered to 90 per cent of patients within five years. Smoking cessation groups are effective for almost all those taking part, but reach only a tiny percentage of those who smoke in an average practice. Charlton *et al.* conclude that GP advice to stop smoking is more cost-effective.

Unfortunately, many aspects of health promotion do not lend themselves to the clinical trial, which is strongly oriented to structured, biologically measurable outcomes. Sarah Cowley (1995) explored two recent attempts to use such a methodology, and concluded that additional approaches to data collection were desirable. Stress management sessions, safety equipment loan schemes, food cooperatives and other health promotion activities, with individuals or communities, do not in general produce clearly measurable outcomes. Theories of behaviour change that start where individuals are, rather than assuming a single common starting point, create difficulties for those who want an ordered evaluation of the outcome of intervention. Interventions that attempt to influence health through manipulating community resources such as the availability of fresh food, cannot by their nature be subject to an analysis that does not also explore the impact of poverty and education on health experience and food use. The banding scheme relies on activity data and morbidity data to establish outcomes. Activity data can only offer proxies for outcome. It will take time to build up a body of morbidity data large enough to demonstrate change.

Child health

A key area of health visiting practice is child health. Community paediatrics has highlighted the importance of identifying children at risk of disease, accident or failure to achieve their full potential, and sees health visitors as key personnel in this task (Hall 1991). Structured schedules of surveillance have been developed to achieve this. They centre around the effective detection of medical and developmental problems, building on the work of the British Paediatric Association's committee, chaired by David Hall, which listed the areas of surveillance that were effective in detecting cases (both sensitive and specific to use the jargon). Health visitors provide an important source in the identification of children in need of protection (Dingwall *et al.* 1983). Many inquiries into child deaths (such as the Cleveland Report 1988) have commented on the importance of health visiting involvement in child protection, and the Children's Act (DoH 1989) has reinforced the definition of the health visitor's role in identifying children with special needs.

All of this has generated increasing concern that the role of health visitors is being restricted within the confines of a biomedical outcome-oriented model. What happens when a health visitor makes routine contact with a family? I visited one family antenatally, and then ten days after the birth of their baby. All seemed well. The baby appeared healthy when examined, the parents were both extremely pleased with their new baby, the father very supportive of the mother. The mother was breastfeeding, with no apparent problems. My next scheduled contact could have been at six weeks at the clinic. However, I was aware of a range of potential social, psychological and biological stresses at this point in the development of the individuals and the family. Babies are constantly changing and developing, not readily predictable; sleep deprivation and hormonal change can each lead to labile emotions; having an ongoing responsibility for the care of the child restricts social interaction outside the family; taking on new roles as parents as well as partners requires negotiation and is stressful; and so on. I therefore said that I would return in a week.

When I returned, I found that both parents looked tired and fraught. The baby had been feeding frequently and was reluctant, it seemed, to settle. My assessment was that there were physiological, psychological and sociological factors involved in the situation. In my interventions I hoped to build up their confidence in their parenting abilities as well as developing a more physiologically appropriate pattern of management.

Over the next few weeks, the feeding settled down to a more manageable pattern. My role was largely reflecting back to the parents, in the light of my analysis, what seemed to be the key issues and, where appropriate, giving them information with which they could make decisions. Having identified their health needs, and not just those of the child, I was attempting to facilitate them in meeting those needs in the context in which they arose, empowering them in developing skills as parents, managing child care and revising their family structure and involvement in society to incorporate a child.

Almost all this activity took place outside the scheduled contacts. It produced no clearly measurable outcome. It required several 'extra' visits of an expensive resource. It is not clear what would have happened if I had accepted the schedule and next made contact at six weeks. Perhaps the family would have presented at the doctor's with their crying, frequently feeding baby and I would have been asked to visit. Perhaps they would have worked out a successful solution on pragmatic grounds. On the criteria of purchasers and paediatricians, largely economic and medical in origin, my activity was unnecessary. Yet, Sarah Cowley's work suggests that most health visiting is done in this grey area of potential risk, identifying and managing health needs, for individuals, families and communities, which go unrecognized by those whose definition of health is more restricted (Cowley, pers. comm.). Meanwhile, many parents, initially content with the level and nature of support received from their health visitors, perceive them as becoming less accessible over time, and focused almost exclusively on 'checking up' – (i.e. surveillance), while the parents themselves identify other needs (Pearson 1995a).

One recurring proposal of those who perceive the essential task of health visitors as surveillance, or see them as an expensive resource, is to implement 'skill-mix'. On the whole, such proposals mean not so much skill-mix as grade-mix, and usually involve the substitution of nursery nurses for one or more health visitors (Cowley 1994). It is believed by those who suggest these schemes that nursery nurses, trained and supervised by health visitors, will be able to undertake routine checks of development and manage simple feeding and sleep problems. Health visitors, while acknowledging the usefulness of such staff, are concerned that they will undertake developmental checks with a more mechanistic approach, perhaps failing to detect early problems in parental health or family dynamics. Their training is in normal development. They have little background in sociology or psychology, and little knowledge of disease processes. They will function mainly in the black and white areas of health or disease, leaving the grey areas undiscovered.

An innovative scheme in Newcastle (Pearson 1995b) sheds light on the process of health visiting from another professional perspective. Working in partnership in an area of deprivation, aiming to benefit families at risk, a health visitor and a social worker are visiting all families with new babies registered with three local practices. At first they visit together, then split up their visits according to what they perceive as the needs of the family. Their records are lengthy, at least partly because of the need to share information. The health visitor records brief information on a wide range of topics, including the child's physical health, feeding and sleeping, the mother's psychological state, housing and any problems with the extended family. The social worker tends to record more detailed in-depth information in one or two focused areas such as housing need or benefit issues. In discussion, the apparent superficiality of the health visiting record is belied by its use as an *aide mémoire* to a relatively complex biopsychosocial analysis. The social worker, whose analysis is more detailed, but mainly derived from psychosocial roots, is gradually adapting to identify a wider range of areas as important, and to recognize the complexity of her analysis as difficult to maintain with a caseload many times the size she is used to. The health visitor is developing a more sophisticated awareness of social need, and learning the value of new perspectives on familiar problems. In working together, each is gaining new dimensions to theory and practice.

Care of the elderly

The final area of practice that I wish to discuss is that of the care of elderly people. Health visitors' involvement in this area has been a small but significant part of their work for many years. With the increasing numbers of frail elderly people in the population, it is likely to continue to be prominent. As with child health, many models to inform practice have stemmed from the medical model of screening for disease, but have tended to be more effective in identifying functional problems. Williamson (1981) has suggested that the process of searching for established disease and resultant disability in order to promote more effective treatment and rehabilitation should be described as 'case-finding'. However, health visitors, rather than searching for disease and disability, are searching for health needs in the broadest biopsychosocial context, and intervening across the same range. Drennan (1986) described a two-stage screening assessment by health visitors, and indicated that the postal questionnaire used in the first stage to identify people at risk of 'socio-medical' problems did not in fact identify people with specific and important problems later uncovered by health visitors, such as 'recent bereavement of very close relatives, marked hearing loss and mobility loss that affected daily living' (Drennan 1986: 211).

Luker (1982) demonstrated that structured intervention by health visitors with elderly people can improve their health status, and that the effects last for some time. However, this study was criticized by Vetter *et al.* (1986) for the limited range of problems in which outcome was evaluated, with no psychological, few social and no environmental problems addressed. They set up a study in two practices in Wales to examine the impact on elderly peoples' health and service use of the employment of health visitors concerned solely with elderly care. One of the health visitors employed appeared to take a very medically oriented approach, confining her work strictly to medical problems and referrals to the GP. The other took a more holistic approach, detecting large numbers of social, environmental and carers' problems, and engaging with a wide variety of other services. Vetter *et al.* concluded that the latter was more effective, and that the health visitor's role was complementary to that of the GP, but stated: 'Nevertheless the effect of this person was to reduce mortality but not disability, though she did improve the quality of life. She also caused a marked increase in provision of services to her caseload' (Vetter *et al.* 1986: 227). In a context that looks closely at costs and outcomes, improved quality of life may be seen as unimportant.

Since these early studies, and others which have questioned the value of a population-based approach to problem detection (McEwan *et al.* 1990), the 1990 GP Contract has made the annual assessment of all patients over seventy-five years of age compulsory for practices. A practice team developing and carrying out its own pattern of assessment for elderly people will find different members emphasizing different aspects. In one practice where I worked, the assessment form was a modified version of a district nursing tool (Poulton 1984), focusing mainly on activities of daily living. I added one question about general well-being. The GPs added questions about mental and emotional state and medication. Each of us appeared to use the same form, but the GPs often took only ten minutes to complete it, whereas I always had difficulty in keeping it under half an hour in the surgery, or longer in the home. The reason for this, in retrospect, may have been that while all members of the primary health care team operate to a greater or lesser extent on a biopsychosocial model of health, GPs tend mainly to be looking for significant biological or functional problems upon which they can act. District nursing priorities are often similar, though they will also explore psychological and social issues for carers. Health visitors, once again, are operating in the grey areas of marginal risk, trying to identify health needs such as social isolation or carer stress which are perhaps currently less measurably important, but which could develop into significant problems.

Biopsychosocial models – integration in practice?

The examples above have demonstrated some ways in which biomedical, psychological and sociological perspectives interlock for health visitors, both in day-to-day practice and at a strategic level. Yet there remains for me, re-reading them, a feeling that the integrated whole has escaped. Perhaps this is because the diversity of ideas on which health visitors draw in day-to-day practice is so great that the integrated whole would resemble a huge patchwork quilt, of which I have described a few squares. At the same time, I am aware that these retrospective analyses suggest a much more ordered and coherent use of theory than is usually the case, for me at least. Textbook theories are usually detailed, and rarely drawn together around cases. Most of my use of theory draws on superficially remembered ideas to illuminate fresh or familiar experiences and suggest strategies for action. Perhaps this is because, as Benner (1984) suggests, much of the analysis takes place unconsciously. It is only usually in recounting one's decision-making process, whether to a student or a colleague, that one attempts to identify what it was precisely that led one to conclude that, for example, marital problems were at the root of a sleep problem, or that a child was at risk. Often one might describe it as a 'gut-feeling'.

Changes and challenges

One of my key themes has been the threat that is posed to an integrated biopsychosocial model in health visiting by an emphasis on measurable outcomes. While biomedical outcome measures are well documented, social, environmental and to some extent psychological outcomes are less clear. Contracts that demand clear measures in order to determine value for money will continue to evaluate health visiting output in terms of contacts made, developmental problems detected and elderly people screened. Areas where outcomes are less clear will increasingly not be included in contracts. The continuing expansion of fundholding general practices may also generate a threat to health visitors' use of an integrated model. As with other forms of contracting, fundholders' business managers will be looking for concrete, measurable outcome areas.

Health visitors' use of an integrated biopsychosocial model may also be threatened by skill-mix. The capacity of an overseeing health visitor to identify warning signs through a third party and to integrate biomedical, psychological and sociological facets appropriately in management plans will be limited. Decreasing numbers of health visitors being trained (*Health Visitors' Journal* 1994) will result in additional pressure to take this route. One area of opportunity that has been briefly alluded to is that of joint working with social services and other non-health agencies. Working across the boundary between health and other agencies facilitates a clearer understanding of the ways in which biomedical, psychological and sociological theories interconnect.

Maybe for health visitors, working on the margins of primary health care will always be our role. Perhaps we need to see our struggle against those who would limit our perspectives to any single direction as an important part of that role. To be most effective, health visitors may need to work across boundaries, whether between primary care and social work or community and authority. In this way, they may develop analyses that help other people to build bridges.

3

Nursing: biopsychosocial care?

John Fulton

Introduction

This chapter is concerned with the question of whether nurses deliver bio-psychosocial care and, if they do, to what extent? It begins by considering the biopsychosocial model within a nursing context. It is suggested that there is a tension between the ideals of practice as taught in nurse education (theory) and the clinical reality of implementing them. This tension will be demonstrated and explored within the chapter by looking in detail at some student nurses' perceptions of the differences between the ideal and real in nursing care in three distinct nursing situations: the care of the dying, care of people who have had cerebral vascular accidents, and the nurse's role with people who have attempted suicide. It will be argued that, in all areas, the provision of psychosocial care is significantly less comprehensive than the provision of physical care.

Nurses themselves have ways to account for not managing to fulfil the broad range of patients' needs. Their accounts highlight the caring associated with their particular practice. But the caring is not of the kind identified by Benner and Wrubel (1989); that is, it is not caring which recognizes the significance of the lived experiences of the client or patient. The nurses' accounts also identify the restraints placed upon them by lack of resources. The chapter puts the argument that the deficit in applying a biopsychosocial model is due not only to a lack of resources in terms of time and staff, but also to nurses' understandable reluctance to connect themselves to care that entails difficult or painful relationships. The education of nursing students in terms of nursing models which may anchor care in the physical domain is also considered as a barrier to nurses delivering biopsychosocial care.

The presence of role models who demonstrate biopsychosocial caring at the 'bedside' may resolve some of the tension between education and practice, but it is concluded that teaching students to be reflexive practitioners may be the best way forward in facilitating nurses in delivering comprehensive biopsychosocial care.

The theory – practice gap

Modern nursing is very strongly influenced by the notion of holistic care. Holism, within nursing, has been equated with the biopsychosocial model. Salvage (1990) has coined the term 'new nursing' to describe the approach, which involves biopsychosocial care based on research findings. In acknowledging and addressing the importance of a wide range of factors involved in care, this approach offers an alternative orientation to that of the medical model and its simplistic equating of patients and the physical conditions they present. The nursing process has been adopted as the vehicle by which effective caring is thought to be implemented.

The nursing process originated in the United States and arose through the increasing professionalization of nursing. The movement towards professionalization included a preoccupation with improving the quality of nursing. Within the nursing process, nursing care is based on assessment, and care is continually monitored and evaluated. The nursing process, by emphasizing that a complete assessment is undertaken of the individual patient's biological, psychological and social needs, and that care is then planned, implemented and evaluated on this basis, becomes a vehicle to ensure the delivery of biopsychosocial care.

Smith (1992) argued that the nursing process is more than a system of documentation, and that it also has the potential to be a philosophy of care. Although Smith does not focus on the term 'biopsychosocial care', the basis of her thesis is that student nurses should be educated in meeting the wide-ranging needs of patients.

As well as providing a structure for the organization of care, the nursing process provides a framework around which nursing curricula are based (Vaughan 1986). Hence, student nurses are taught according to the biopsychosocial model and in this context a great deal of emphasis is placed on the holistic care of patients and the curricular subjects reflect this. For example, as well as being taught basic physiology, student nurses are also taught psychology and sociology.

There is a tension between what is taught and its implementation in practice (Hunt 1974; Bendall 1975). Ford and Walsh (1994) point out that there is a widespread 'dislike' of the nursing process. They base their argument on the vast amount of material appearing in the nursing press that criticizes the nursing process, maintaining that it stems from a top-down approach. One may conclude that the nursing process is not whole-heartedly embraced by practitioners. This raises the question as to whether the seeming dislike of the nursing process reflects a more fundamental disagreement with a biopsychosocial philosophy of care.

To help to address the question of whether practitioners are in philosophical disagreement with the biopsychosocial model, or whether there are other very good reasons for nurses' failure to embrace the model, I will draw upon my own research. The research sought to access the experience of student nurses as they were being socialized into a biopsychosocial approach to the delivery of nursing care. Of central interest to me was an exploration of how biopsychosocial philosophy was translated into practice through the eyes of student nurses. Student nurses were chosen as they were exposed both to the ideal in the educational situation, and the reality of clinical practice in close coupled sequences. Therefore, they were thought to be in an appropriate position from which to judge the translation of the ideal into reality.

As well as taking accounts from student nurses, the research involved a careful selection of nursing areas. Every nursing area differs in the emphasis that needs to be placed on the particular elements of the biopsychosocial model. Within the study, three particular areas of nursing were selected as an appropriate means of exploring the commitment ward-based nurses gave to biopsychosocial caring: nursing with individuals suffering from a cerebral vascular accident (CVA), nursing with dying patients and nursing with people who had attempted suicide. The initial physical crisis of the CVA victim requires a physical, biologically based approach, although nursing the person through recovery requires all three elements of the biopsychosocial model to be given roughly equal weight. Care of the dying requires a high level of skill in applying biopsychosocial concepts throughout, while the care of the individual who has attempted suicide is a situation where psychosocial needs are more prominent. In addition, the 'illness' trajectory for the persons who had attempted suicide was important. For example, it might be seen as a crucial part of biopsychosocial nursing to understand something of the circumstances that led up to the person attempting to take his or her own life.

The following section summarizes themes that emerged from exploring student nurses' experience of being in the different nursing areas. It should be noted that the theory presented is substantive. It is relevant only to in-patient nursing and cannot be generalized to all nursing care, or care by other disciplines in relation to the biopsychosocial model. To do so, a broader sweep of nursing practice (e.g. including community nursing, differently graded nursing staff, different professionals, etc.) would have been necessary.

Exploring the tension between theory and practice

The question, posed above, concerned whether nurses are philosophically opposed to the biopsychosocial model or are constrained in some ways from implementing it. A theoretical discussion is needed to address the question adequately. The discussion interweaves themes emergent from my study. Overall, it attempts to show how nurses establish boundaries that delimit the extent of caring in accordance with their emotional capabilities and perceived professional competence.

In the study, nurses looking after patients in all three groups were very connected to physical caring. For example, all students emphasized the excellent physical care of dying patients: 'The care was very, very good. If they needed to be turned every two hours, then they were . . . everything was geared towards the patient'. However, the level of physical care varied across nursing areas. For example, the emphasis was placed very much on basic physical care needs when working with CVA patients, whereas there was a feeling that the primary needs of terminally ill patients were somewhat different:

> If it was my mother I'd want it better. I'd want, like in the morning you do under the arms, chest, bottom, you never wash under the feet. Well I don't, you don't have the time. It's shameful really. Hair – you get the hair done. It's a boost to get your hair done with rollers in it, and they're lucky to get that done once a week or every two weeks. And bowels, there's a lot of constipation here.

The technical aspects of care, or more accurately rehabilitation, were mainly delivered by physiotherapists, and were not, in many instances, followed through by nurses:

> The physios go on a lot about keeping their fingers straight, keeping their foot lying in a certain position – it doesn't happen. When I came here at first a nurse said: 'What are you doing?'

The student nurses in the study seemed aware of the gulf between ideal and real caring. All the students could articulate the care the patients should receive, but acknowledged that this did not seem to happen in reality. The student nurses constructed accounts that rationalized the theory–practice gap. For example, in relation to patients with CVA, they gave accounts of care deficits in terms of resource issues:

> Up to a point the care is good, I think you learn in school the proper way – to sit with everyone whose had a stroke to have a meal, to turn the plate, to remind them whatever side it's on and to give them all their aids. I don't think there's always someone available to do this. You don't have time. There's so much to do and so few staff to do it – and some things aren't seen as that important. I'd like to find time for odd

things, like the patients' psychological well-being, just to keep them happy and content, because I'm pretty sure I wouldn't like to sit in a chair all day.

Resource issues were also a very real, and justified, concern. Staffing levels vary from situation to situation. With increased patient through-put, nurses in both medical and rehabilitation settings acknowledged the constraints there were to delivering any kind of integrative care. Nurses are often expected to deal with a range of patients with diverse needs, often coupled with situations perceived as varying significantly in terms of available levels of support and back-up. Constraints in time often mean they can only really attend to the physical, in the sense of daily living needs, as these are (visibly) the most pressing and immediate the patients have. But resource issues were not the sole reason for not meeting psychosocial needs.

The 'matter-of-factness' of physical caring made it easier to provide than psychosocial care. It seemed as though the nurses could cope provided boundaries were in place around the patient; that is, they were categorized as needing physical care. The nurses' need for boundaries is illustrated by their concern over 'becoming involved with' patients.

Many nurses commented that they did not realize how entangled they could become with the patients. In order to prevent becoming emotionally 'caught up', such patients were categorized by nurses as individuals requiring predominantly *physical* care. This was particularly easy when age and/or physical status intervened. For example, both age and level of consciousness provided a boundary to emotional caring. Those patients who could not be categorized as having reached the end of their natural life, or who were aware of their situation, caused the nurses more distress. As two student nurses put it, in referring to dying patients:

These people were, you know older – I've never come across anyone who was younger.

The first lady I looked after was distressed. If they are in a coma it's all right, but one lady knew she was dying and was distressed. It was horrible.

Under conditions when physical caring boundaries were not well defined, the nurses tried to redefine them or erect new ones. One example of this was marginalization. This finding is in keeping with research into nursing spanning the last thirty years. For example, Glaser and Strauss (1965) found dying patients marginalized and shut off from the mainstream of ward life. Menzies (1970) identified strategies and 'blocking', behaviours used to prevent nurses discussing the particular concerns and needs of patients beyond the level of social niceties.

Menzies (1970) investigated ways in which care is organized and delivered at a ward level. She found that work was organized in such a way as to prevent the nurse from becoming too involved with the patient. Thus, the organization of work served as a defence against the anxiety that such an involvement could produce. The management of specific episodes is 'laid down' in nursing tradition and so has a life of its own. In other words, ways of dealing with particular categories of patients have become institutionalized. Menzies argued that these institutional defences prevented individual nurses from confronting and working through their feelings and thereby developing mechanisms for dealing with the feelings that the patients could induce in the nurses. The student nurses in the present study commented, that in many instances, dying patients were marginalized through the routine ward procedure of being closeted in cubicles:

> They always put them [dying patients] in a cubicle off the ward. I think that's terrible 'cause the patient knew: 'Oh God, I've come to a cubicle . . .'. They were just there to die off the ward. I think the nurses didn't have to go and see them. It'd have been nicer for the patient to have been in a bay – the other patients cope better than we give them credit for.

Another form of marginalization was keeping contact with patients and relatives at a superficial, social level. Boundaries are often set through the pattern of communication. For example, the involvement of the family was commented on to a much greater degree in nursing the group of dying patients, and families were allowed and encouraged to become involved in the care of patients. However, the interaction with families was usually at the level of 'everyday' social intercourse, rather than being focused on their, or their relative's, emotional needs: 'All the relatives we've had have been quite nice. We get to know quite a few families'.

So far, I have argued that boundaries were established around caring which kept families' psychosocial needs in abeyance. Nurses did not become involved or intervene in a systematic way in order to satisfy these needs. The concern about being emotionally caught up was also evident in reports about caring for individual dying patients:

> . . . there was one ward I got really involved with the family . . . after she died I went to the funeral and everything and after that I thought I'm never going to another patient's funeral. It was so upsetting.

Another means to re-establish boundaries around physical caring was to define the unmet needs of the patient as the responsibility of other health personnel. This strategy was particularly evident in nursing with people who had attempted suicide. Nurses were careful to distinguish psychiatry as outside their role, or competence. It was clearly perceived that it was the role of the psychiatrist to deal with people who had attempted suicide. The patients were seen as boarders on the ward, accessing its hotel services. It was not perceived as part of the nurse's role to deal with these emotional needs. The role was limited to physical caring, with psychological and social needs being largely ignored:

> We didn't have much to do with them.

> We were unsure how to deal with them.

> The attitude displayed towards them – it's your fault.

> We didn't even have the time to say: 'Why did you take it? Do you want to talk about it?' The psychiatrist did that sort of thing.

However, unlike with the patients with CVA or dying patients, individuals who had attempted suicide were not seen as being particularly disadvantaged by having their physical care prioritized. There was not the same perception that there was a yawning gap between the real and the ideal. The student nurses largely seemed to be in agreement with the *status quo* that these individuals were boarders on the ward and not in need of therapeutic intervention. The implication is that, for this particular group of patients, a biopsychosocial philosophy of care was not valued. However, such a statement is an over-generalization, as the next section argues.

Attempting to close the theory–practice gap

So far, I have implied that nurses establish or re-establish boundaries that preclude psychosocial caring as a means to protect their own emotions. Yet, many nurses did realize that their patients had needs beyond the physical, engaged with those patients around those needs, and worked towards meeting them. In so doing, they were, effectively, closing the theory–practice gap. For example, there *were* nurses who found time to be with people who had attempted suicide:

> They were usually pushed to one side – the stance being 'silly bugger' taking their own life, we're trying to save other people's lives. However, on one ward they did sit down and talk to them. There was this young girl, if she got upset they'd take her into a room, sit down and talk to her. The care was really good.

The quotation indicates that some nurses were not against the philosophy of the biopsychosocial model, in relation to caring for people who had attempted suicide. Nurses who spent time dealing with the patients' emotional needs provided a strong role model, and powerful learning experience for the students: 'I actually sat in on a session with one staff. It was really good. I thought "you've [*I've*] taken the wrong approach all along".' While a good role model may have beneficial effects, the comments of another student nurse illustrate the lack of modelling of good practice:

You talk about stages of dying and talk about helping patients through, but that's not done. I find it really difficult to deal with someone who is dying and not having any guidance – we hear about it in class but I don't see people deal with it, the stages.

As the student nurses in this study were exposed to a variety of environments, one can conclude that biopsychosocial caring was not demonstrated in a systematic way. It would, therefore, be difficult for nurses to build and develop their skills pre- and post-qualifying.

Without a consistent and systematic role model of psychosocial care, the adoption and development of the application of the biopsychosocial model would seem to be left to chance. Smith (1992) argued that the lived ward experience of student nurses is crucial in their development, and very influential in developing their future approach to nursing care. She noted that the role of the ward sister/charge nurse is instrumental in setting a context for biopsychosocial caring, in that the particular experience of student nurses can determine whether they model themselves as people-oriented or task-oriented nurses. People-oriented ward sisters emphasize the emotional aspects of care. A ward sister or charge nurse concerned with caring in a broad sense opens up the opportunity for the implementation of the biopsychosocial model because he or she is not preoccupied with the physical aspects of care. The nurse in charge of the ward, and the team ethos he or she promotes, may therefore provide a narrowing of the educational–practice gap.

However, while clinical staff may provide role models for the students, they may not be trained educators and may not be aware of the students' educational preparation for the clinical environment; they therefore cannot always extend their role to clinical teaching (Reynolds 1990; Clifford 1993). Ferguson and Jinks (1994: 692), in considering the theory–practice divide, suggested that '. . . integration will only be achieved if those staff responsible for classroom teaching are also closely involved in clinical supervision of students'. The availability in the clinical arena of a nurse tutor may also provide a role model for good practice: '. . . tutors should be competent to practice as first level nurses, have in-depth knowledge of nursing and be in touch with the realities of practice at macro and micro levels. In addition, they should act as facilitators of good practice and as a resource for staff' (ibid., p.693).

Having nursing tutors in the clinical environment may therefore assist students to apply what they are learning. However, what they are learning may not necessarily facilitate biopsychosocial care. A number of nursing models have been devised and are taught in the classroom situation. These models are also referred to as conceptual frameworks (Riehl and Roy 1980), or as an attempt to put the meat on the bones of the nursing process (Aggleton and Chalmers 1987). Models have been devised by drawing on theories from the physical and social sciences to provide a framework within which the nurse may make a meaningful assessment, plan the care, and be aware of what interventions to make and how and what to evaluate (Aggleton and Chalmers 1987). There are several nursing models, perhaps the most popular of which in Britain is the Activities of Daily Living model (Roper *et al*. 1980). This model requires the nurse to assess the patient in terms of the activities relating to his or her daily living activities.

Webb (1990) has suggested that nursing models may provide a basis for structuring student learning if they are combined into nursing curricula. For Smith (1982), the inclusion of nursing models into curricula would enable teaching to reflect current practice and make the resulting nursing care more holistic.

While this implies that nursing models may help to bridge the theory–practice gap, Miller (1985) pointed out that nursing models may exacerbate the theory–practice divide. Although such models aspire to encompass biopsychosocial understandings, the primacy of physical caring is evident. The ease with which physical care is undertaken may be sustained and even justified by the dominance of physical aspects within nursing models. Thus at one level (the physical) there may be consensus between theory and practice, but this consensus inhibits the links at other levels (the psychological and the social). Nursing models that claim to incorporate biopsychosocial understandings may nevertheless fail to facilitate the provision of holistic care. I turn now to a more detailed analysis of 'caring' in order to assess whether caring can be defined in such a way as to provide a foil against which the biopsychosocial model is more likely to be implemented.

Caring

There are two aspects to caring: one concerned with the person-oriented aspects of patient care and another, theoretically based, concerned with technical and skilled aspects of care. Dunlop (1986) suggested that there should be a science *of* caring as well as a science *for* caring. That is, the meaning that the experience of caring has for the nurse and patient is defined as the science *of* caring, and the knowledge and skills necessary to deliver effective care can be defined as the science *for* caring.

Care, whether holistic or not, was a recurrent theme across all nursing areas. All of the nurses spoke of their activities in terms of caring, and it was apparent that they saw their actions as having meaning for themselves and for their patients. They felt they were caring for people by doing something for them that would have a positive effect on them, that would make them, in no matter how small a way, feel better. Watson (1979) viewed caring as almost synonymous with nursing. Benner and Wrubel (1989) have defined the primacy of caring as being connected to, and concerned about, patients, so that a context is set in which the application of knowledge and techniques becomes practicable. However, in being connected, the nurse must necessarily encounter emotional involvement:

Caring . . . means that persons . . . matter to people . . . *caring* is used appropriately to describe a wide range of involvements, from romantic love to parental love to friendship, from caring about one's garden to caring about one's work to caring for *and about* [my emphasis] one's patients.

(Benner and Wrubel 1989: 1)

In the study reported here, of particular interest is the boundaries nurses constructed around their delivery of care, and the ways in which they were not allowed to develop their own coping strategies but rather had to adopt the strategies of the environment in which they were working. As Menzies (1970) suggested, this prevents student nurses from developing their own coping strategies and thereby perpetuates the system where the patient's psychological and social needs may be ignored. In this scenario, it is difficult to argue that the primacy of caring, as described by Benner and Wrubel (1989), was present, or that the nurses were practising in a way consistent with a science *of* caring.

The nurses' practice also lacked evidence of a science *for* caring. Thus, while all the student nurses emphasized the importance of being with the patient and ensuring that nursing interventions had a positive effect on the patient, the care often lacked the technical dimension in terms of skilled interventions. The student nurse requires the theoretical knowledge important to the delivery of biopsychosocial care and the consistent monitoring of the development of these skills. In other words, an adequate science for caring is a prerequisite *for* the delivery of biopsychosocial care.

Conclusion

Holism in nursing is defined as equivalent to the biopsychosocial model of caring, as encompassed in the nursing process. The nursing process is not popular with nurses at the bedside. There is tension between education and practice which is appreciated by student nurses who are exposed to the ideal and the real in close coupled sequences of training and ward experience.

An examination of three disparate groups of patients, in terms of their care needs, indicated that the biopsychosocial model was not systematically followed. Nurses tended to focus on the patients' physical needs. Nurses are not in opposition to biopsychosocial care, but find it difficult to implement. Resource issues are one form of constraint, but these are less important than the emotional consequences of psychosocial caring for nurses. Nurses find ways in which to erect boundaries between themselves and their patients in order to protect their emotions.

However, some nurses did attend to the biopsychosocial needs of their patients, which also indicated their agreement with a biopsychosocial philosophy of care. These nurses are good role models for less experienced, or able, practitioners. Without role models who demonstrate biopsychosocial caring, the gap between theory and practice may be self-perpetuating.

The findings of this study are in keeping with the reports of researchers in the 1980s, such as Orton (1981), Fretwell (1982) and Ogier (1986), all of whom identified good and bad learning environments and saw the ward sister as crucial in creating the emotional climate of the ward. The inclusion of nurse tutors at a clinical level may provide a role model for students that goes beyond that of ward sisters, in that tutors can create a bridge with the classroom environment. Yet the models of nursing as taught in the classroom may not instil the biopsychosocial understandings in nurses which they are deemed to incorporate.

An interesting way of examining nursing is in terms of the science *of* caring and the science *for* caring (Dunlop 1986). The present research would suggest that both are important, as we need to understand both the meaning of care – and nursing care in particular – and how the theory and skills necessary for that care can be best taught to student nurses. The role of educational experience is vital in preparing nurses with competencies to deliver care in complex and dynamic situations (Schön 1987). In order to prepare students adequately to deliver biopsychosocial care, encouragement to reflect upon their practice, utilizing existing theories and their experiences, will need to be given.

4

Negotiating boundaries: reconciling differences in mental health teamwork

Chris Stevenson and Phil Barker

Introduction

This chapter discusses the complex of 'world views' that distinguish disciplines, in terms of how these world views 'own' different languages and definitions of mental illness. The languages and definitions comprise a disciplinary 'grammar' as a pattern of putting words together in order to explain the world. The ways in which disciplines with different world views explain and 'deal with' mental health problems will also be explored. The chapter will consider how the professionals involved in multidisciplinary teamwork might find ways of working collaboratively rather than being in conflict. It will be suggested that a negotiation of boundaries between disciplines will be necessary if effective multidisciplinary teamwork is to develop. The chapter draws extensively on the experience of the authors in practice settings.

World views

It has become commonplace to refer to 'mental health problems' as a politically correct synonym for what previously might have been called mental *illness* or *disorder* ('emotionally different' is only one of a number of other alternative descriptors of the same phenomenon (see Beard and Cerf 1992)). However, such linguistic developments, which can easily be dismissed as a passing 'faddism', belie more serious issues concerning the role of language in the definition and explanation of abstract phenomena such as 'mental health'. Such problems reflect emotional or 'psychical' disturbance, which is, by and large, invisible. The discrete terminology defines, for example, symptoms and specific disorders, and the general language of the social sciences talks about, for example, personality and mental state. Such terminology and language may be more tangible than the phenomena to which they refer. Mental health problems may be vague and abstract, but the language of psychiatry and the social sciences provide a security of understanding that may well be misleading.

The way mental health problems are defined and explained derives from the attitudes and value systems of the various disciplines that have, traditionally, come into contact with the 'sufferers' of such problems. Indeed, the language of psychiatry and psychology has become embedded in the everyday vernacular, and has become a means by which people describe and explain their everyday experiences. Although controversy and conflict have characterized the whole history of psychiatry and the social sciences, such terminology, and the many values and philosophies upon which it is based, is only now beginning to be questioned seriously.

Much of this conflict derives from the different forms of explanation used by the various health or social service disciplines. Psychiatric physicians are likely, by and large, to favour a broadly biomedical explanation of the person's problems and to offer biophysical forms of treatment. Clinical psychologists are more likely to invoke 'psychic' or non-physical explanations, and to offer 'treatment' based on psychodynamic or cognitive theories of the human condition. Social workers, by contrast, are likely to favour an explanation that acknowledges the influence and potential usefulness of the environment and social context.

Sheppard (1991) considered the theoretical orientation of social workers and community psychiatric nurses (CPNs) involved in mental health teams, and found that social workers were oriented towards social science understandings and the interpretation of actions into meanings, whereas the focus of the CPNs was on mental health. The two professional groups:

> . . . define clients with meanings particular to their profession . . .
> Social workers' concern is with psychosocial problems or needs . . .
> Nursing differs from social work in its emphasis on health. Their biopsychosocial orientation is more ambitious than that of social work.
>
> (Sheppard 1991: 24–25)

The different disciplines are, increasingly, thrown together within multidisciplinary teams (MDTs) that provide 'community care', and that are becoming increasingly popular (Toseland *et al.* 1986). The teams are often the point of entry for referrals of people defined as having mental health problems. Often a 'referral meeting' is held at which the various professionals in the team bid to take on specific cases. For example, a referral from a GP requesting some counselling may lead to one or more professional 'volunteering' to take on the case. The bid is driven by a complex interaction of variables (e.g. current caseload size, perceived competence, etc.). The success or otherwise of the bid results from the negotiated protocols that the team are applying. In other words, the upshot of the necessity of working together is the invention of ways of collaborating with one another, despite differences in theoretical understanding. It is to these differences that we now turn.

Levels of explanation

When a mental health problem is identified, a wide range of explanations of the phenomenon is possible. Taking the example of schizophrenia, the phenomena ('picture', presentation, symptomatology, etc.) are open to interpretation on a number of levels. Each of these levels purports to 'explain' the distress experienced by the individual. For example, the biological explanation might be that the problem derives from a disturbance in neurotransmitter activity, whereas a psychological explanation is that the problem involves difficulties in the ability to process information. These individualistic explanations are very different from explanations that see the individual in his or her social context; for example, a social structural position connects schizophrenia to the race/class/power structure of society, whereas an interpersonal analysis views the 'schizophrenic' presentation as a natural function of the person's relationships with significant others. A social constructionist stance entails the idea that the 'schizophrenic' individual is created and sustained through the stories which he or she and significant others choose to tell about problems.

This list is not exhaustive. It does, however, suggest the diversity of explanations possible, each reflecting a different level of analysis.

The nature of explanations

In principle, the explanations noted above are simply ways of making sense of events or phenomena. No one level of analysis and interpretation is, necessarily, better than another. Since professionals from different disciplines use such analyses to make different 'sense' of problems like schizophrenia, there is a potential for conflict. Birch (1995), referring to the description and treatment of schizophrenia, notes that the community of psychiatric workers does not usually subscribe to a shared single story:

> All too often the big issue for psychiatric workers around schizophrenia is what to do about the Bad Guys. It's easy for one camp to believe in the Bad Guys when they hear a client report that they have been

advised: 'You have an imbalance of the chemicals in your brain'. They are sure that, as advice narratives go, this is not just philosophically suspect, but also a recipe for disempowerment. Equally it's easy for the other camp to believe in the Bad Guys when they hear a practitioner say: 'I don't make use of the construct "schizophrenia".' This camp finds such a position obtuse or callous.

(Birch 1995: 226)

The emergent disciplinary boundaries define and distinguish the different professions in terms of which service they offer and how they relate to the other professional disciplines. One would hope that, in practice, professionals would rarely try to impose an overarching explanation of the problem. Instead, the diversity of explanations, or interpretations, would be viewed as contributing towards a menu of services, each of which is the responsibility of the different disciplines. As a result, for example, it would be the psychiatrist's job to prescribe the medication, the psychologist's job to test for memory impairment, and the nurse's job to engage in a meaningful interpersonal relationship with the person in order to address any 'problem of living'. A successful multidisciplinary team, McGrath (1991) noted, would have shared aims, but distinct roles and expertise, each member of the team being responsible for delivering a discrete service and differing markedly from other team members in skill or experience in offering such a service.

Underlying a fondness for multiple explanations, however, lies a strong attachment to dualism. Each level of explanation compartmentalizes 'reality'. Mental states are seen as separate from biology. They are not reducible to any form of materialism. There is a strong, post-Enlightenment tradition in Western society of celebrating materialism over 'mentalism'. Within the sphere of health explanations, biology is more valid than subjective experience in understanding mental health problems.

Perceived power and the management of explanations

Foucault (1975) argued that health settings involve knowledge/power hierarchies. In Western societies, those disciplines that can demonstrate knowledge based on scientific research are seen as having 'better' knowledge. Biomedicine claims such a scientific knowledge base. Consequently, there is a pervasive belief, both in lay and in professional circles, that doctors have precedence over others in acting on their theories. Much medical practice is pragmatic and heavily influenced by the attitudes and values of the physician. Indeed, Charlton (1993) has advocated a breadth of academic experience for the trainee medic in order that they have a broader perspective on problems. In this sense, it might be more appropriate to talk of the 'art' of medicine, which though based loosely on a range of other sciences – such as physiology and biochemistry – is based also on the humanities. Traditionally, however, physicians have tended to operate from the position that medicine *per se* is a science. As a result, Bowling (1983) argued that the medical profession assumes dominance over 'semi-professions' which have less theoretical underpinning.

The perception of status differences can be a constraining factor on multidisciplinary working. A classic illustration is the 'multidisciplinary' ward round. Information that is collected by the nursing staff, psychologist, social worker and occupational therapist is conveyed to the consultant psychiatrist, who may choose to use, or dispense with, the information given when making a decision about the person's 'care'. The decision is part and parcel of the physician's 'clinical judgement'. Typically, the other professionals within the 'team' would accede to the psychiatrist's decision. This is not an example of multidisciplinary teamwork but, rather, is an illustration of medical hegemony and a resultant clear pecking order. Fiorelli (1988) has argued that because of the inherent organizational hierarchy and diverse professional cultures, it is deeply naive to think that multidisciplinary meetings operate in an egalitarian fashion. Little appears to have changed since McIntosh and Dingwall (1978) noted that primary health care teams could not operate effectively because the power and generalized expertise claimed by physicians was an obstacle to professionals from other disciplines collaborating on equal terms. A contemporary example is the status of the 'fund-holding GP'. Here a GP has full control over the health care budget for a defined sector of the community – that is, the patients within his or her practice. The GP has the power, therefore, to determine which clinical services are offered within the practice, or 'bought in' from external agencies, such as hospital clinics. The GP also has the power to influence the role of professionals from other disciplines (e.g. practice nurses, clinical psychologists, counsellors) by determining what are the needs of the patient population and, consequently, 'buying' the services he or she thinks are required to meet those needs.

However, when community care is implemented, the power issues between disciplines are brought into sharp focus, because they are required to work together to provide comprehensive packages of care. For example, one of the authors has been involved with a project where a multidisciplinary team approach to risk assessment is being developed. The usual medical authority is not taken for granted. In this real world of practice, the risk assessment will involve community psychiatric nurses and medics *conjointly* making judgements about whether someone is suicidal, assessing individual needs and matching the person's needs to services available. The conjoint assessment and decision making will be possible because there is an agreed interdisciplinary assessment format and a shared philosophy of care that will be formalized through inter-professional training. It differs from existing practice where the psychiatrist tends to have the 'last word'. Without some shared philosophy about the nature of mental health problems and the ways in which help can be organized, it is difficult to see how the team could function.

Yet, the practice referred to is not customary, and the more usual arrangement is that of medical dominance. Perhaps the 'worst case scenario is that the lead-clinician, who adopts the dominant (parental) role will encourage submissive (childlike) behaviour in other members of the team' (Berne 1968). Where MDTs are characterized by strife and disharmony, they invariably bear a striking similarity to families in conflict. For example, alliances between professionals are similar to those between family members, as both can have the function of disempowering other people within the system (Haley 1963). A question is begged of whether or not health professionals, who accede to medical dominance at an overt level, covertly think that their explanation (or world view) is better than those of others. Do the different disciplines involved in MDTs simply 'play along' with the power game, perhaps inadvertently reinforcing the relationship transactions that are characteristic of the power scenario? Where one professional (such as the physician) is responsible for determining the 'need' and the 'necessary service', the participating disciplines may all too easily adopt passive (or irresponsible) positions. Furnham *et al.* (1981) suggest that professionals are inclined to think of their own profession in a more positive light than others. Each sees his or her own practice as being more broadly based. In terms of practice, the psychotherapist may concede to the psychiatrist's prescription (or world view), but gets on with what he or she covertly perceives as the real work, for example talking to the person.

The generic worker?

If specific professionals within the team are defined narrowly, in terms of their role and/or function, this might limit the 'creative' development of the service. Paterson (1992) considered that team members have simultaneously to balance the allegiances with their own professional group with the knowledge that individual professions do not have an exclusive right to any body of knowledge, and the need to share common goals. Iles and Auluck (1990) noted that the areas of social work practice involving teamwork are increasing and this can raise tensions at both theoretical and practice levels. If the view is taken that the social worker, for example, is the only person who addresses the family context, or issues concerning housing, this *may* define the professional too narrowly. The social worker may feel that he or she has little scope for development. In his or her absence, the other team members may feel unable to address the 'social work' issues. Working within more flexible boundaries however offers the team the potential to manage situations in a variety of ways.

While some skills may be the focus of one professional, other areas may be shared by many professionals. For example, a professional of one discipline may take on a function that is usually associated with another discipline: the psychiatrist may take on a small psychotherapy caseload; the psychiatric nurse may adopt *both* a psychological approach to depression (e.g. cognitive therapy) and practise systemic family therapy. In subscribing to both therapeutic approaches, the nurse is holding both individualistically and socially oriented theories; and the social worker may provide the escort and transport for a client attending a depot injection clinic, thereby intervening on a social level in order to facilitate biointervention. Such a shift of professional emphasis connotes a move from the task orientation associated traditionally with different professions, to the most practical and flexible means of providing a service driven by the actual needs of the clientele. The marked flexibility of professional roles and the degree of blurring or overlap between one professional group and another, are increasingly features of many MDTs (Kane 1975).

At one level, the professional may draw on the separate levels of explanation outlined above, as justification for practising some approach to care or treatment that is markedly different from that taken by others of the same discipline. Conversely, he or she may claim that there is a common characteristic underpinning all of the professional activities, and that this unifying factor is the *raison d'être* of the whole team. Carson (1994) noted that 'caring', in its broadest sense, is shared across disciplines. There may be a common characteristic underpinning explanations of problematic behaviour. For example, although the psychiatric nurse, who practises different forms of therapy, may acknowledge that there is something special in the act of conversing with the person (the non-specific treatment factor), the viewpoint may also be taken (in parallel) that all problems, whether social, biological or psychological, are in some way connected to the need for self-expression in an appropriate environment. The team negotiates not only the relationships among its various members, but also their orchestrated relationship with the client body. User empowerment through recent legislation, for example the *Patients' Charter* (DoH 1991a), has led to a shift in the generally held perception that professionals are all powerful. It may be axiomatic that the flexibility required of the 'team' to be able to respond appropriately to the 'client body' needs to be reflected, internally, in a flexible relationship structure among the team membership. Referring back to Birch's (1995) review of professional positions on schizophrenia helps us to see the value of flexibility and respect between professionals:

If life is text, this covert, and sometimes overt, sniping between opposing camps of professional helpers is inseparable from 'schizophrenia' in the late twentieth century. A discourse amongst the camps which was more respectful would inevitably become a discourse about a different schizophrenia, and could be a discourse more useful to those who seek our views on how they might find a more coherent story for their lives.

(Birch 1995: 227)

Social construction of need

A more complex analysis of the means by which professionals negotiate a working relationship concerns the active co-construction of meaning by individual practitioners in a specific agency. People with mental health problems rarely 'know' the nature of their needs when they make contact with the service. Indeed, it is only through the process of dialogue with the team members that the nature of the problem, and what 'needs' to be done, emerges. It might be naive, however, to assume that the team members uncover – or, in some sense, discover – the problem. It might be more appropriate to adopt the 'world view' that through active dialogue both parties define something that, previously, was not known.

Social constructionism is the position that 'who we are' is constructed by the interaction we have with others. Berger and Luckmann (1967) addressed the dualist tension between the individual and the social by suggesting that realities are constructed through a complex circular interplay between self and society. The person is both defined by, and defines, the society in which he or she lives.

'Mutuality' defines the variety of roles required of the professional and the different contexts within which the service of the team is offered. In the context of a mental health agency, the roles that professionals of specific disciplines take might also be constructed through interaction with one another. As the roles are constructed, so they will in turn define the agency, and so on. For example, the social worker may take on cases for cognitive therapy, the occupational therapist might give advice about medication. The extended roles are locally agreed and are not constrained by the customary disciplinary constraints. Very complex agreements may then be set up. For example, the agency may be adapted to include a supervision system whereby the 'beginner', taking on a new role, has access to support, and the expert maintains some control. As the 'beginner' becomes more skilled, an alternative form of supervision may emerge. For example, both the authors have experienced 'peer supervision' when a sharing of views about 'cases' can take place without any imperative to take on advice, which often arises within an hierarchical arrangement.

Beyond social constructionist theory

Stainton Rogers (1991) reviewed attempts (e.g. social constructionism) to bring together the individual and the social as explanations. According to

Henriques *et al.* (1984) and Doise (1986), a 'democratic fusion' of theories is impossible. They are different levels of discourse. Social constructionist theory is inadequate in addressing the tension between the individual and the social. It is simply a way of papering over the duality that exists. In the same way, it is an inadequate means for professionals to paper over the cracks that exist between their respective views of the world.

Kuhn (1962) described paradigm shifts in which the old model is over-thrown by the new. However, the extent to which a revolution in theoretical development occurs is debatable. At any one time, many contradictory theories about the world seem to compete, as in the example of the alterna-tive theories about schizophrenia articulated above. In Bernstein's (1983: 46) view, much of the difficulty concerning theoretical knowledge involves 'the persistent claim that it is science and science alone that is the measure of reality, knowledge and truth'. Within the context of a mental health service, science is, of course, the underpinning science of biomedicine. Press (1980) has coined the term 'synpatricity' to describe the wealth of theories about a social phenomenon. Although the different theories compete, they manage to co-exist in parallel. The truth may well be that, not only is reality socially constructed, but also that knowledge *per se* is problematic and contested (Lather 1984). Given the synpatricity of theory, it may be appropriate to consider the value of 'alternative paradigms' as the stabilizers for a social phenomenon such as the MDT. From this perspective, *alternative* para-digms are the ideational structures that portray humans as beings who generate different forms through which they hope to understand and repre-sent the world they inhabit. It involves taking a view of mind and know-ledge that does not entail the idea that there is only one way in which we can know our world and a single observable reality (Eisner 1990).

Conclusion

There is a complex of world views on mental health problems, each with its particular language set and explanatory form. Each explanation is simply one way of making sense of mental health problems, and no one level of analysis and interpretation is necessarily better than another. However, as different disciplines favour a specific explanation, there is the potential for conflict to arise.

In practice, the professionals of different disciplines may find a way to negotiate shared goals, but with discrete roles. However, such an arrange-ment is underpinned by dualism, a likely concomitant of which is that materialism is celebrated over 'mentalism'. Consequently, those disciplines attracted to materialist explanations are likely to take precedence in what is essentially a knowledge/power hierarchy. The result is a clear professional 'pecking order' that does not facilitate multidisciplinary working. There are many scenarios in which multidisciplinary working is not truly operating. For example, it may be that professionals simply 'pay lip service' to the world view of others while getting on with what they define as the 'real work'.

Yet there are examples, particularly in community settings, when disciplines apparently work together successfully in a flattened hierarchy. This type of working may be underpinned by different local arrangements. For example, MDT working, which adopts a generic work ethic, neutralizes professional power bases. Role flexibility can be rationalized through the idea that professionals inevitably 'care'. When flexibility and respect for others' understandings of the world are embraced, it is possible for professionals to co-construct their identities and so set up locally based, complex agreements in order to deliver quality care.

However, for some authors, co-creating professional roles is simply a way of covering over the tensions between world views. The whole endeavour of finding common ground is based on the assumption that competing, but co-existing, theories are problematic. An alternative description is that a range of theories enriches the ecology of ideas about mental health problems.

5

Multidisciplinary child protection and interdisciplinary perspectives on child abuse and neglect

Neil Cooper and Alison McInnes

Introduction

This chapter considers how theoretical models aimed at understanding child abuse are applied within child protection, and whether or not such models can be integrated in practice. The chapter will briefly describe the major role of multidisciplinary work in child protection and how the interdisciplinary understandings of child mistreatment interrelate with multidisciplinary action. With respect to this chapter, a multidisciplinary approach is considered to be the joint and coordinated action of several agencies, such as professionals belonging to social services, health and legal organizations; interdisciplinary understandings refers to academic disciplines such as biology, psychology and sociology.

The chapter evolved from one author (McInnes) working and researching within child protection in the social services domain, and the other (Cooper) researching into the psychology of child protection. Working within social work and working with children has coloured how events have been perceived by ourselves and how the information gathered and discussed in this chapter is considered.

First, the range of professionals potentially involved in child protection will be considered, and it will be shown that child protection policy has emphasized that agencies must work together. The different perspectives on understanding child abuse and neglect will then be considered, and it will be shown that models of child abuse have been developed that draw upon biological, psychological and social aspects of the phenomenon. It will be argued that while theories have been developed, and there is the potential for understanding child abuse from within an integrated model, working definitions are largely descriptive and that professional practice utilizes academic understandings of the problem to facilitate the management of abuse at an individual case level. It will be demonstrated that an integrated model of abuse is impossible to employ in current practice. In order to integrate the different theoretical positions, it will be suggested that the professionals involved in child abuse must become experts, with the term 'expert' being defined in a way that may allow all practitioners to aspire to expertise.

Multidisciplinary child protection work

The agencies with statutory responsibilities for child protection are local authorities (through social services departments), the National Society for the Prevention of Cruelty to Children (NSPCC) and the police. The remaining professional contributions to child protection are not statutory; however, their role within child protection may be related to other statutory responsibilities, and includes a wide array of professionals working within diverse situations, such as health visitors, school nurses, midwives, paediatricians, general practitioners, psychiatrists, casualty doctors, police surgeons, teachers, educational psychologists, local authority solicitors and probation officers. At a local level, Area Child Protection Committees (ACPCs), consisting of a multidisciplinary management team, are responsible, among other things, for developing and reviewing guidelines and for interdisciplinary training.

The professions that may be involved in child protection therefore have different roles and responsibilities in relation to children. It is between these professions that strong pressure for cooperation and coordination exists at both practice and policy levels, as a multidisciplinary approach has been widely advocated in the management of child abuse. A multidisciplinary approach, however, is a relatively recent development.

Following the professional identification of child abuse, initially labelled 'baby battering' (Kempe *et al.* 1962), societal awareness of child abuse as a social problem requiring professional input began to develop. Multidisciplinary management started to evolve as the roles and responsibilities of different agencies began to be established, and these have been continuously refined, especially in response to public inquires into child deaths, which occurred throughout the 1970s and 1980s. These cases centred around inadequate parenting and the physical abuse of children, while more recent inquires have focused much more on the organization of inter-agency work (Cleveland Report 1988; Orkney Report 1992). While the focus of reports has shifted from individual children to agency actions during major investigations, they have continued to re-emphasize the importance of multidisciplinary work and emphasize working together. The Department of Health guidelines, aptly titled *Working Together* (1991b), in conjunction with the Children's Act (1989), provide the basis for professional action in which multidisciplinary cooperation is central. The preface to the *Working Together* document stated that it is 'well established that good child protection work requires good inter-agency co-operation' (DoH 1991b: iii). This ideal is constantly reaffirmed throughout the document.

While policy documents stress multidisciplinary work as good working practice, there are many inherent difficulties in such work. The professionals required to work together in child protection operate within dynamic systems between the state and society. They have different responsibilities, operate within diverse organizational backgrounds with different working practices, professional cultures, organizational hierarchies between and within professions, and they often operate in child protection at a time of high anxiety. Such issues can lead to problems in multidisciplinary work (Dingwall *et al.* 1983; French 1984; Weightman 1988). The mechanisms of multidisciplinary meetings and decision making may produce conflict as well as cooperation.

These problems are acknowledged to some degree in policy documents:

> . . . co-operation and collaboration between different agencies is a difficult and complex process, particularly in an area of work like child protection in which policy and practice are constantly developing to absorb new ideas acquired through experience, research and innovative practice. All agencies concerned with the care of children are aware of the need to adapt and change in response to the growth of knowledge and understanding.
>
> (DoH 1991b: 5)

While this emphasizes the need for professionals to adapt to new knowledge, it does not consider what type of knowledge. If professionals are required to work together in child protection, they need to share meanings. However, many different models have been postulated to explain child abuse and neglect. Professionals working within different agencies may subscribe to different forms of knowledge related to such practical aspects as their organizational structures, the training ethos, historical development, methods of intervention, working practices and relationships with clients.

Interdisciplinary understanding of child abuse and neglect

Corby (1989) identified seven major approaches in the explanation and understanding of child abuse: sociobiological, psychodynamic, behaviourist, family dysfunction, sociological, feminist and children's rights. Corby suggested that the theoretical areas move along a scale 'which starts with biologically based approaches, moves on to psychological and social theories and ends with a focus on political and philosophical considerations' (p.30).

The more philosophical aspects concerning children's rights lead to broad conceptualizations of child abuse, as illustrated by Gil (1979). Loney (1989) suggested that the concern with the child's development expressed through broad definitions allows for the development of an holistic approach to child abuse. However, such broad considerations of what may constitute abuse are difficult to relate to practice issues at an individual case level, and therefore the more practical theoretical approaches that attempt to explain child abuse are usually utilized by practitioners. These approaches are based upon biology, psychology and sociology. The theoretical base used by professionals therefore reflects biopsychosocial understandings, and an integration of approaches may be linked with a biopsychosocial view. However, an integrated model has yet to be developed. Why might this be?

While authors such as Gil (1979) indicate that abuse may be any action or inaction that prevents a child reaching his or her full potential, practice documents tend to split abuse up into typologies, typically physical, sexual, emotional and neglect. This categorization of forms of abuse, while practical, is an evolutionary result of the rediscovery of abuse. While the theoretical perspectives suggested above appear to imply a number of ways of viewing abuse, the theoretical dimensions have not always been presented concurrently. Rather than initially thinking about how the theoretical underpinnings of understanding child abuse may form an integrated biopsychosocial model, it makes more sense to consider how the different understandings have been utilized to frame and understand child abuse since the 1960s. It can be considered that different models have developed in tandem with the 'discovery' and definition of different forms of abuse, as Table 5.1 shows.

In the 1960s, a pathological paradigm was evident in which the individual pathology of the abuser was the focus of concern. The medical model was utilized within psychiatric understandings, with the general concept of personality being that of stable and measurable traits:

> Psychiatric factors are probably of prime importance in the pathogenesis of the disorder . . . Parents who inflict abuse on their children do not necessarily have psychopathic or sociopathic personalities or come from borderline socioeconomic groups, although most published cases have been in these categories.
>
> (Kempe *et al.* 1962: 20)

The abusive tendencies that Kempe considered have been compared to simplistic notions such as the nineteenth-century idea of the 'criminal mind' (Montgomery 1982). If child abuse is regarded as a disease, this implies that medicine can diagnose abuse and formulate cures that focus upon individualized treatment (Pelton 1978; Frude 1980). The medical model used in

Table 5.1 Emergence of different theoretical perspectives in the 'rediscovery' of child abuse.

	Decade			
	1960s	*1970s*	*1980s*	*1990s*
Context	Physical abuse	Physical abuse/ neglect	Sexual abuse	Ritual/ organized abuse
	'Baby battering' discovered	Child death inquiries	Cleveland 'crisis'	Allegations in Nottingham, Bradford and Orkney
Emergent explanatory framework	Medical/ psychiatric	Sociological/ psychodynamic	Feminist	Cultural/ symbolic

child abuse focused on the individual and prevented an appreciation of the social and cultural factors that create a context for abuse. Despite the medical model being untenable when applied to social aspects implied in abuse, it has continued to underpin professional action.

Throughout the 1970s, the concept of stable personality traits was contested within psychology and an increasing emphasis on situations occurred (Pervin 1978). The pathological reasons for child abuse were becoming minimized, and sociological sources of stress, such as single parenting and lack of social support networks, were implicated in abuse, and the links between socioeconomic position and abuse were reluctantly accepted (Gillham 1994). Such a perspective, linking social conditions with child health, identified child abuse as a social problem with an increasing remit for the involvement of social workers rather than medical practitioners. Social workers, however, needed models in which to practise at an individual case level.

Psychodynamic understandings became critical in the development of explanations for child abuse; for example, the work of Bowlby in the examination of early bonding relationships led to a practical concern with family dynamics and parent–child relationships. The utilization of such a model provided practitioners with a theoretical justification for action and also provided an aim for action in relation to individual children. In basing practice on the model, the professionals also removed the individual case from its social and cultural context, and continued the concept that 'treatment' could be directed at 'the problem'.

In the 1970s and 1980s, sexual abuse was rediscovered and constructed into a social problem. While physical abuse was rediscovered in medicine via radiography (Pfohl 1976), and the development of medical expertise in establishing the presence of abuse was important throughout the inquiries of the 1970s and early 1980s, medical conclusions regarding sexual abuse are much more difficult to substantiate (Hobbs and Wynne 1989). The medical model therefore had difficulty in explaining sexual abuse from a theoretical perspective, and also had practical problems in establishing signs and symptoms for the 'condition'. As the medical model could explain the actions of parents in relation to physical abuse, much of the policy and procedures had also been formulated in terms of physical abuse and neglect, and were ineffective for the investigation of sexual abuse (Wattam 1992). Feminist literature created the main understanding of sexual abuse and placed responsibility for abuse with gender relationships at a structural level. The development of a feminist discourse offered social and individual intervention strategies (Waldby *et al.* 1989). Utilizing such an approach also places more emphasis on symbolic aspects of relationships and interactions.

The 'discovery' of 'organized' and 'ritual' abuse in the 1990s again produced a challenge to professional perspectives. The comprehension of this form of abuse requires social and cultural understandings, and it is no accident that the 'expert' brought in to investigate was an academic anthropologist with previous experience of symbolic understandings of violence in other societies, whereas previous investigations into child abuse incidents had been conducted by prominent legal professionals. Cultural aspects of abuse had been understood, but more often cultural awareness referred to action within individual cases involving people from ethnic backgrounds rather than an awareness of the British culture.

The theories utilized within professional discourse, therefore, lead to different conceptualizations of the problem and consequently to different solutions. Sociocultural and feminist explanations demand social change at a structural level, psychological theories seek change in individuals and families, and medical models implicate individual treatment as a route through which change may be made. While academic understanding of child abuse and neglect is largely disciplinary, practitioners often use interdisciplinary knowledge (Gallmeier and Bonner 1992). All the different approaches and theoretical orientations considered above assist in explaining child abuse and neglect. However, each approach has limitations in its application. Could these approaches be integrated?

Garbarino (1977) suggested an ecological approach to child abuse in an attempt to cope with the complex human systems that produce it. Garbarino suggested that child abuse is a point on a continuum of caregiver–child relations and therefore quantitatively different from non-abusive relationships. For Garbarino, two conditions are necessary for abusive relationships to develop: culturally sanctioned disciplinary actions towards children that justify abuse, and a lack of social support for parents. Garbarino's model, while not explicitly a biopsychosocial model, considers adaptation to the environment as an interacting system. However, such an approach is not holistic, as it does not allow for the individual; there is the risk of making use of the ecological fallacy, in which large-scale data are drawn upon erroneously to draw conclusions about individuals. Belsky (1980) went on to consider this integration of perspectives through ecology and conceptualized child abuse as:

> . . . a social-psychological phenomenon that is multiply determined by forces at work in the individual (ontogenetic development) and the family (the microsystem), as well as in the community (the exosystem) and the culture (the macro system) in which both the individual and the family are embedded.
>
> (Belsky 1980: 320)

Following Belsky's approach, Kaufman and Zigler (1992) developed a concept of risk factors and protective factors based upon the different areas of concern.

The phenomenon of child abuse may therefore be understandable within the same dialogue of knowledge. Practice, however, maintains distinctions between the different forms of abuse, and neglects those theories that indicate a broad conceptualization of the problem.

As indicated in Chapter 6, the professional definition of what constitutes abuse and neglect are often commonsense-type statements, and in practice the application of the definition is left to individual practitioners (Herzberger 1988). A homogeneous theory would include broad aspects, such as neighbourhood safety, which practitioners might find difficult to work with at an individual client or family level. So, for example, if a consideration of the socioeconomic situation is integrated into a general model, this leads to change at a structural level rather than at an individual level. Theories that have been very influential in child abuse offer the professional an individual framework. Bowlby's work on maternal deprivation and the importance of early experience, for example, was an integrating force in the early 1970s in which professionals could construct ideas about childhood and parenting that related directly to their work (Hendricks 1990). Bowlby's concepts also gave practitioners something tangible to work with at the individual and family level, in that they could consider relationships within the family and work to improve them. Practitioners in their everyday work are oriented towards working with individuals and families; this means that models utilized by practitioners are more oriented towards individual action and change, and are therefore somewhat anchored in the medical model. The neglect of the political role of professionalism has parallels in more common health issues (Blaxter 1983). If professional models continue to function from a basis in biomedicine, what sustains this position?

Sustaining models of abuse

Hallett (1993) considered that the issues of how clients are perceived, local factors and professional values will affect what is labelled as child abuse by a professional. Despite this, Hallett (1993: 143) suggested that 'There is fairly widespread agreement amongst the professionals that, in general, cases referred to or identified by the relevant agencies as child protection cases are appropriate . . . that the thresholds of intervention being applied are broadly acceptable'.

It can be seen that the professional perspectives have a foundation in the medical understanding of child abuse and all consequent models refer back to this initial conceptualization. Garbarino (1977: 721) suggested:

> From its beginning as a field of inquiry child abuse has been dominated by the clinically defined area of pathology . . . professionals and public alike have defined child abuse as qualitatively different from normal caregiver–child relations. This 'medical model', which concentrates on 'kinds of people' theories in many ways represents a paradigmatic re-sponse to deviance.

Figure 5.1 demonstrates that multi-agency work shares some common values and understandings. The focus of the work, however, becomes what is required by the professionals to suit a particular case situation; that is, the theories drawn upon are amorphous and allow for the individualized 'man-agement' of the problem. It does not matter if the prevailing management system is medical or not; the way in which the system is anchored within the medical approach maintains action at the individual case level.

The management of the problem feeds back into the construction of the problem together with other influences, such as the media reporting of investigations and research reports. This feedback mechanism will main-tain, for a certain period of time, a preferred management approach to child abuse. The perceived importance of professional input into child protection may be related to this prevailing approach. So, for example, while medical input to child protection is very important in many cases, GPs have repeat-edly been identified as being poor attendees at child protection case con-ferences (Harris 1991; Lea-Cox and Hall 1991). While practical issues such as surgery times may account for some absences, Simpson *et al.* (1994) conclude that low attendance is due to the low priority GPs attach to child protection conferences. Given the statutory importance of social services, and the shift away from the biomedical management of child abuse, GPs' poor attendance may be a response to the GP's role within child protection being marginalized by both organizational and ideological pressures. At-tachment to one form of management leads to particular forms of training being perceived as necessary. Once professional training in child abuse is oriented around a particular ethos, this may in turn encourage more re-sources, more training and more clients to be dealt with. The successful

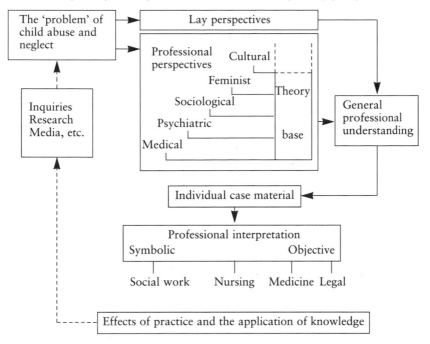

Figure 5.1 The process of accumulation of explanatory models of abuse into general professional understanding and practice.

management of clients perpetuates the perceived model of child abuse, and reinforces the professionals' knowledge and ability to intervene and at the same time may push other professionals to the periphery.

While the different theoretical models of child abuse combine to create a general professional understanding, there is some differentiation in the way that the knowledge and beliefs are applied. Professionals such as lawyers, police officers and doctors operate around 'facts' and there is little consideration of the symbolic functions used to understand family life by such professionals as social workers (Valentine 1994). Social workers and the police are at loggerheads because the allegations of abuse expose a fundamental difference in the types of evidence they are looking for. Social workers are charged with finding victims and ensuring that they are safe, whereas the police have a primary interest in finding the perpetrator(s) of the abuse. Here are two cultures of evidence that through intolerance and misunderstanding can find no common theme (O'Sullivan 1990).

Thomas (1994), however, indicated that some acts in relation to children are criminal and dealt with through the law, where objectivity and factual evidence from lawyers and police officers are appropriate and unavoidable. These examples indicate the real tensions that exist in the way in which professions involved in child protection draw upon and utilize information.

Members of different professions will interpret the same case material differently along the symbolic – objective continuum. This does not mean that social workers are not objective, but that the way they interpret the material allows for the inclusion of symbolic representation to a much greater degree than other professionals. For example, the recognition that a child is rarely taken out of a high chair may be based upon observations from several visits by staff from different agencies. This information may mean different things to the different professionals. The social worker, for example, may view the constraint of the high chair as having adverse developmental effects and as reflecting the parent–child relationship; that is, the child in the high chair is symbolic of the relationship. The medical professionals may share these symbolic ideas, but they will not enter into the discourse. The medical practitioner will be more concerned with the physical symptoms of being restrained in a chair. The health visitor will share the symbolic concepts, too, but will be concerned with how the restriction on mobility is affecting development, and may link how the child is doing compared with other children of the same age through reference to the 'normal' milestones of development. While the input of each professional adds information to the case, the information will also help to create a collective map of understanding, or schema which guides intervention. Child protection workers may be overloaded with information relevant to any particular case (Dingwall 1986), and schemata allow professionals to simplify reality (Fiske and Taylor 1984).

Because of the diversity of interpretative stances derived from the same general understanding of the issues, statements made in inter-agency forums may have one meaning for the individual uttering it and different meanings for the other professionals in accordance with their underlying interpretations and input regarding the specific case. In any given situation in which abuse is suspected, professionals may attempt to obtain certain forms of information to assist in their interpretation of the situation from within their professional view. All professions however remain constrained by the need to perceive the situation in a way that can be managed by intervention at the individual case level. The interpretations which emerge as the basis for action will result from professional negotiation. The theoretical understanding used by professionals is therefore not eclectic, but rather amorphous. That is, the theory underpinning practice depends upon the context in which a particular case of child abuse or neglect occurs and what action appears most appropriate to manage the situation.

Different professional groups will therefore possess different narratives of what abuse is and how best it should be managed, despite having access to the same general pool of knowledge and beliefs. Professional discourses, the way in which professionals talk about child abuse, are incommensurable, but find common ground in action. Child abuse gets managed. It is the need to manage child abuse that sustains models of abuse. Despite knowledge being available regarding social and cultural aspects of child abuse, professional practice is based on biological and psychological models. Can multidisciplinary child protection operate with a more holistic approach based on interdisciplinary knowledge?

Multidisciplinary and interdisciplinary integration – impossible or undesirable?

> It is, we believe, a recipe for disaster for professionals ever to become enmeshed in a particular theory . . . that it becomes 'taken for granted' . . . We believe that single minded models of the 'problem', its 'detection' and its 'solution' help to create the pressure under which child abuse professionals work.
>
> (Stainton Rogers and Stainton Rogers 1989: 50)

The nature of multi-agency work – the public disgrace when things go wrong, the resource implications of child protection work and the personal anxieties of individual professionals – may draw professional workers deeper into specific and familiar interpretations to exonerate their actions.

Teamwork could be advocated to allow the team to share responsibility (as described in Chapter 4). A team approach, however, may create local elites of specialists, in which knowledge may be perceived as esoteric, and the everyday identification and management of abuse may be feared by those professionals not involved in the team. Rather than a team approach, a close working multidisciplinary partnership is required, not only at the practice level, but also at the management level.

Perhaps a more successful way of ensuring successful multidisciplinary work would be to encourage professionals to be holistic. Hallett (1993: 151) considered several advantages of multi-agency work, one of which is to increase the capacity 'to deliver comprehensive holistic services'. The form of holism is not, however, defined. Holistic practitioners must maintain their work orientation, fulfil their statutory obligations and duties. However, they need also to reflect on practice and not become entrenched in any one model. We suggest that holistic practitioners are also 'experts'.

Professional 'expert' knowledge may be vital in particular areas of child protection. In relation to courtroom evidence, Williams (1993: 713) states that:

> The position of experts is a special one, as they are particularly privileged in law. All witnesses are, of course, entitled to state the facts as they know them. However, only experts are then allowed to go onto give an opinion in evidence. The court can, and may well, give great weight to this opinion.
>
> (Williams 1993: 713)

Wattam (1992), however, demonstrates how experts can be used in court proceedings to validate a particular interpretation of 'facts'.

A claim to expertise based upon experience with particular forms of abuse and an up-to-date knowledge of the literature means that few practitioners are regarded as expert (Myers 1993). However, in discussing expert witnesses, Myers indicated that some form of generalized accepted opinion is usually involved in identifying an expert: 'The important issue is whether the expert's opinion is based on types of information typically relied on by other experts . . .' (ibid., p.177). This suggests that all experts refer back to a common pool of professional knowledge. Furniss (1991) considered that while experts are employed within legal cases, child abuse is bigger than any one individual's skills and knowledge: 'we will only be able to face the multiprofessional challenge of child sexual abuse if we maintain our respect for our own specific professional skills and trust our own professional expertise' (p.110).

For Furniss (1991: 261), being expert means being able to 'respect the expertise, the skill and the responsibilities of fellow professionals'. We would suggest that experts in this sense are holistic professionals, open-minded, aware of their own values, and aware of the models of abuse which operate in professional circles and society. Professionals from different agencies therefore do not need to practise from a similar theoretical background, as this could lead to professional 'greyness'. Differences in approach should be celebrated and actualized, and used for the benefit of the service user in the delivery of holistic care.

While the current system of child protection allows for crisis intervention and management, and holistic care may be an achievable goal in this area, a broader conceptualization of child abuse and child protection, which is the inevitable result of reflecting on professional action and interpretation, demands that wider social and cultural issues be addressed. If professionals could act on social and cultural aspects of child abuse, as they are acknowledged in theoretical models of abuse, the potential for holistic child protection management would be much greater than at the crisis level.

Part 2

Lay perspectives

Introduction

This part of the book looks at lay perspectives and how they both share and challenge the biopsychosocial understandings in professional models. Following from Chapter 5, which focused on professional understandings of child abuse, Neil Cooper and Alison McInnes consider how lay understandings of abuse map onto professional models. The chapter reflects the positions of both authors, who do not agree on all points; the differences in perspective and the debates that developed in the process of writing the chapter in many ways mirror the child protection issues discussed, with their inherent tensions and contradictions.

The chapter considers how the different forms of explanation that make up the biopsychosocial model can be utilized by professionals and lay people to arrive at different constructions of the same situation. By discussing this in relation to child abuse and protection, it is demonstrated that the different levels of explanation have moral implications. For example, a father who hits his child when socially stressed may be seen as less morally reprehensible than a father who sexually abuses his teenage daughter. However, an understanding of this behaviour may be based upon biological interpretations, which imply a degree of determinism. On this argument, it could be considered that the sexually abusive father's actions are biological impulses beyond his control; therefore, it could be argued that as not all stressed parents hit their children, the sexually abusive father is less culpable. This complex area illustrates the conflicts and contradictions that arise in the use of the biopsychosocial model when different explanations provide different but equally valid justifications for child abuse.

Chapter 6 concludes by suggesting that the biopsychosocial understandings used by adults may obscure the explanations used by children, and it is argued that a more complete understanding of children's conceptualizations of abuse may create the conditions that will allow the deterministic notions of the biopsychosocial model to be transcended.

Nigel Watson continues this consideration of lay perspectives in Chapter 7, where he notes that health promotion involves a very wide range of occupational groups and that health promotion specialists coordinate the activities of other professionals. Nigel suggests that health promotion originates in a socioecological conception of health that is characterized by a movement away from disease or medical models. He provides a convincing argument for the deconstruction of the medical model of health by foregrounding lay beliefs. An alternative, holistic model of health promotion necessarily includes physical, mental, emotional, social, spiritual and societal aspects. The difference between a biomedical and holistic model is their different emphases on the physical. However, Nigel points out that the tensions that exist between biological essentialism and social relativism will soon emerge in health promotion practice.

Implicit in Nigel's chapter is the position that a biopsychosocial model, if applied by health professionals and/or health promotion experts, would not take account of lay beliefs. The narrative offered by professionals influenced by the biopsychosocial or any other health model may simply not match the narrative favoured by lay people. For example, the range of stories about a health or ill-health behaviour, even if each one incorporates biopsychosocial elements, is potentially vast. Take two different biopsychosocial accounts of smoking, for example: the first states that anxiety is reduced by the physical effects of nicotine at a synaptic level; the second states that 'nerves' are reduced by the effect of inhaling deeply during smoking.

It is argued that if health promotion is to be effective, then lay beliefs must be given a prominent place in health discourse. If not, the complex meanings that people attach to certain behaviours and the social and moral constraints by which they live will mean that a restrictive health promotion model will simply fail.

In Chapter 8, Shaun Kinghorn and Richard Gamlin review the conversion of lay beliefs to action through a demand for complementary therapies. They use their extensive experience of hospice work to inform their analysis of the individual merits of conventional biomedicine and complementary approaches to cancer. The authors are not naive to the tensions between medicine and complementary therapy and they set out some of the likely sources of conflict. A major question that they address is whether the two positions can be reconciled in order to provide the best possible cancer care for those living 'in the shadow of the crab'.

Shaun and Richard deconstruct the popularly held view that a cure for cancer through biological intervention is close at hand. They provide both lay and research-based evidence that many medical treatments, although able to increase life expectancy, are unsatisfactory because of the associated physical discomfort.

Shaun and Richard argue that people need 'magic as well as medicine' but that magic and medicine lie in an uneasy relationship with one another. Conventional cancer care is based on systematic scientific inquiry; complementary therapy is typically justified by anecdotal knowledge that is seen as 'softer' in Western society. They have different knowledge bases. Shaun and Richard argue for rigorous scientific trials to assess the effectiveness of complementary therapies. Yet they also indicate that new paradigm research, which is an alternative approach to inquiry, can complement orthodox scientific research in its quest for a cure. They demonstrate the dilemma that arises when approaches with different underpinning philosophies are a foil for one another.

One reason for the dilemma is the failure of biomedicine to adapt to embrace complementary approaches. Shaun and Richard argue that the consumers of care themselves may be a force for changing the current dominant biomedical view of cancer. Taking a nursing perspective, they give a sense of the dilemma nurses have in balancing lay demands for complementary therapy against a concern for the efficacy of such therapies. The situation is complicated further by organizational/resource issues and uncertainty over the competence of complementary therapists.

A solution offered by Shaun and Richard is similar to one that Chris Stevenson and Phil Barker note in Chapter 4, the suggestion that each practitioner working in a multidisciplinary team should take on a clearly defined role. The role includes offering an aspect of the complementary approach which matches best with disciplinary training. However, even when the provision of complementary approaches is divided between disciplines, Richard and Shaun recognize that practice is enacted in domains where professional guidelines are sometimes 'patchy' or contradictory. Providers of care will be obliged to develop policies that define the range of practice and overcome ambiguity in the face of lay demand.

Whereas Shaun and Richard argue for a 'model' of cancer care that balances both the biomedical approach and more holistically oriented, complementary therapies, Glynis Hale takes a more radical stance to models of caring in Chapter 9. Taking a social constructionist perspective towards bereavement and grief, she deconstructs how professional models create 'normalized' grief reactions. Glynis argues that any treatment models based upon biopsychosocial understandings, while claiming to be holistic in nature, constrain the way in which researchers and practitioners may regard bereavement. For Glynis, the increasing development and sophistication of such models will continue to confine professional understandings. She demonstrates that narrow professional understandings of grief also affect lay people who may not experience the 'normal' patterns proscribed by professionals. Professional models are also used to guide practice and affect how professionals interact with clients in situations such as counselling. Glynis advocates that sophisticated models of grief that constrain understanding should be abandoned for a more open approach to practice that allows for individual narratives of the experience of grief to be shared. She argues that such a position may leave the practitioners without the safety net of professional models, and suggests that this is an area requiring further exploration.

6

Lay understandings on child abuse and neglect: utilizing explanations

Neil Cooper and Alison McInnes

Introduction

This chapter argues that the professional understandings of child abuse that orient around multifaceted causes as represented in the biopsychosocial model may be shared by lay adults and children. The tensions inherent within the biopsychosocial model may be used to give alternative conceptualizations of why child abuse occurs within professional and lay interaction. Understandings about abuse are related to strategies to manage it. This chapter will demonstrate that the authoritative explanations of child abuse are situated within professional discourse, which leads to professional intervention being the only viable alternative for its management.

How lay views are heard in the child protection process will be demonstrated by looking at the child protection case conference. It will be shown that child protection case management is often *not* negotiated between professionals, parents and children, and the conference can be regarded as a stage upon which the positions of the different perspectives are acted out.

Finally, the implications for the biopsychosocial model provoked by the consideration of lay views will be considered. It will be argued that the concept of client empowerment is not necessarily helpful, and that lay views provoke alternative ways of 'intervention'. An example will be given of the way in which work with families may be seen as child protection.

Explaining abuse and managing protection

Two questions can be considered important in this area. First, what constitutes abuse? And second, why does it occur? In relation to the first question, it can be considered that as child abuse is socially constructed, what constitutes abuse will be related to the social and cultural factors operating within an individual's environment. Child abuse is a moral issue and professionals make moral judgements about cases:

> . . . subjective judgements are made about whether certain behaviours or outcomes constitute child abuse. These are affected by many factors, including social class and ethnicity of the children and family; workers' frames of reference and personal values, local levels of awareness and local operational procedures.
>
> (Hallett 1993: 143)

All individuals, whether lay persons or professionals, will have their own views as to what constitutes abuse. However, due to a shared cultural experience there will be some commonalties. For example, we live in a society that finds the physical punishment of children to some degree acceptable and this acceptance of physical punishment means that physical abuse can be conceptualized:

> It seems as if society must develop through stages of awareness over a considerable period of time, before true acceptance is achieved. And it appears to be fairly self-evident that physical abuse is the easiest form of abuse to acknowledge and accept. We have over the years condoned a certain amount of physical abuse towards children.
>
> (Johnson 1990: 42)

Gil (1979) considered child abuse from the perspective of the rights of the child and proposed a broad definition of abuse:

> . . . any act of commission or omission by individuals, institutions, or society as a whole . . . which deprive children of equal rights or liberties and/or interfere with their optimal development, constitute by definition, abusive or neglectful acts or conditions.
>
> (Gil 1979: 4)

This definition is based upon a philosophical stance and is so expansive that it can include so many behaviours and attitudes in relation to children that it may be difficult to apply in practice.

Professionals who are involved in child protection tend to utilize more discrete definitions of abuse which are able to distinguish between different types of abuse, and such definitions are often found in policy and procedural guidelines. These definitions of abuse and neglect appear to be 'common sense evidentiary expressions which legislators feel no reasonable person could misinterpret' (Belsey 1993: 45). This suggests that a 'reasonable' person can know the difference between normal childrearing and abusive situations.

However, it may be considered that professional action taken to increase understanding and 'accuracy' may be unnecessary and abusive in itself. Professionals are aware of the potential for child protection to be abusive. Furniss (1991) commented that professional networks in themselves may be abusing, as children get drawn into institutional conflicts; this recognizes that professionals operate in a social world. Other actions may appear less understandable to lay people.

Levitt, for example, in considering diagnostic techniques, suggested that a doctor may perform an anal examination 'that includes the penetration of the boy's anus by the physician's gloved and lubricated examining finger . . . The physician can . . . ask him to define whether the touch was at the anal opening or actually inside the anal opening as the finger enters the anus' (Levitt 1990: 236). Levitt suggested that this allows the boy to compare the investigative sensation with the sensations of abuse. This is indicative of the biological being emphasized as representing the 'truth' of abuse. This action may, however, be seen as abusive in itself. Swift 'dawn raids' by the child protection team may also be perceived as being emotionally disturbing for children, demonstrating that a 'social' response may be no better than a 'biological' approach in child protection, with the rationale behind such actions being considered ill-informed. Despite their subscription to models of child abuse based upon academic research, the actual actions carried out by professionals can be difficult to understand.

Explanation in child abuse is not just an adult arena. There is a developing children's rights discourse which affects many areas of society (Franklin 1989), and how children's views and rights may be incorporated into child protection is receiving increasing attention (Freeman 1983; Cloke and Davies 1995). Freeman identified the protectionist and liberationist schools of thought regarding the rights of children. The former is well entrenched in our legal system, but the liberationists take a more radical stance with the view that children as far as possible should have the same rights as adults. Since the Cleveland Report (1988), the view that children should be heard has frequently been advocated, and agencies have attempted to create a climate in which children are listened to. This appears to endorse the liberationist viewpoint. The development of the liberationist discourse is, however, inhibited somewhat by adult perspectives that control the definition and management of child abuse. As adults are seen to possess a more developed morality than children, it is assumed that they are more aware of what is right and wrong. Adults, however, may also be considered to be more knowledgeable than children, and therefore that adult explanations are also more complex. So, for example, the concept that an abuser may be biologically driven to an abusive action (such as through inherited aggressiveness) moderates the moral aspects. Such biological explanations may not be available to a child, who may refer to more social explanations.

The definition of abuse may be subtly different between children and adults. In a survey commissioned by Barnardos (1995), it was shown that adults were concerned about crime, bullying, violence and drugs. While children's views reflected some adults' concerns regarding violence and bullying, 57 per cent worried that their parents might divorce. This demonstrates the differences in the adult and child worlds. The effects of divorce were seen by children to be detrimental to them and consequently they could be conceptualized as abuse. While adults acknowledge that divorce may be painful for children, divorce does not enter into their discourse of child abuse.

In a similar way, children may fear the consequences of professional intervention in an abusive situation due to the disruption this may bring to a family. In interviewing children about their experiences of child abuse investigations, Taylor *et al.* (1993: 163) reported the following response from a child: 'I just wanted to be a normal family. When the police got involved, I was frightened they would put my dad in prison'.

There are therefore tensions and alliances between the professionals, lay adults and children in the way in which they may draw upon biological, social and psychological understandings. These explanations may underpin stories that are constructed around abuse.

While the stories may be shared, the meaning of the stories may be different for each individual or each group. Lay adult and child stories may overlap in drawing upon a social aspect, such as sharing the view that strangers are more dangerous than those people known to a child, although the meaning of the word 'stranger' may be different for children and adults. Sometimes the meanings of the stories may be shared across groups, so that the professional and adult lay perspective may share some understandings due to a shared perception originating within the media and due to shared experiences in childhood. Professionals and lay adults may also share psychological reactions to abuse. Finally, all three groups may share views that originate in the operation of shared cultural understandings and wider social forces.

In many ways, child abuse is no different from other aspects of health and illness. Radley (1994: 19) suggested that:

> . . . health and illness are also dependent upon the social context in which sickness occurs and in which it is treated. We cannot assume that words like 'ache', 'pain' or 'doctor' – or even 'health' and 'illness' for that matter – refer to things that remain the same wherever and whenever they are applied.

As in the treatment of health problems, having a particular explanation for abuse will lead to a particular strategy for management. It can be considered that child protection is controlled by professional understandings of abuse, while the lay views of adults and children have a limited effect upon the child protection arena.

Despite being able to draw upon academic understandings of child abuse, Corby (1987) indicated that within multi-agency decision making there is little direct reference to literature and research. The ways in which professionals use subjective judgements and rules of thumb in child protection practice have been identified. Dingwall *et al.* (1983), for example, considered that professionals often use the 'rule of optimism' in child abuse investigations. One aspect of this rule is the concept of 'natural love', the idea that parents love their children because they are *their* children. This has echoes in the sentiments within lay discourse that children are 'safe' within the family. Underpinning such sentiments may be a fusion of social and biological explanations as suggested by sociobiology, which draws upon genetics in order to explain aspects of human action (Wilson 1975). From a sociobiological viewpoint, people are more willing to help those to whom they are more closely genetically related. Thus physically harming one's own children becomes illogical, and may be explained through psychological processes (the parent must be disturbed).

A sociobiological analysis also suggests that sexual abuse by non-genetically linked relatives (such as step-parents) is more easily understood. A stepfather suspected of sexual abuse, who expresses that he cares for his stepdaughter (individual processes), may be regarded with suspicion by both professionals and other lay people alike who infer that he could not care for her as if she was his biological daughter. Peace (1991) indicated that sexual abuse is seen by professionals and the public as being more criminal than other forms of abuse, and that sexual abuse crossed a moral boundary. This may explain the public 'uproar' that followed the events in Cleveland in 1988, in which the notion that children could be sexually abused by their parents produced 'a wave of protest against the idea that such things could happen' (La Fontaine 1990: 7). While a parent may sympathize with another parent who has hit a child in particularly stressful circumstances, due to the moral dimension of sexual abuse, an explanation which focuses on individual (psychological) factors may be favoured when such abuse is suspected. Those suspected of sexual abuse however, may offer explanations which are more oriented around situational factors. This shows that conflicting views of a situation may be constructed regarding abuse.

The explanations prevalent in lay understandings may be married with professional discourse. Morrison *et al.* (1987), writing from experience of professional reluctance to accept sexual abuse, considered twenty 'myths' that may prevail in professional meetings, including: 'Boys are never sexually abused' (p.9), and 'It was a stranger, and a one off event – so there's no probability of serious damage' (p.11). This indicates that professionals, like lay people, may consider situations based on simplistic notions rather than on explicit research and theoretical understanding. Why should these stories exist?

Child abuse is a very complex phenomenon. Simplistic notions can be very powerful and can become perceived as 'facts' – accepted knowledge about 'how the world is'. For example, with respect to the 'cycle of abuse', Kaufman and Zigler (1987: 186) considered that 'The belief that abused children are likely to become abusive parents is widely accepted by professionals and lay people alike . . . Despite the popularity of this belief there is a paucity of empirical evidence'. Comprehending abusive situations in this way may have a protectionist function for adult society by serving as a defence to minimize the deliberateness of abusers' behaviour, and to focus upon abusers repeating what they learned in childhood (Kelly 1992).

Other common perceptions about abuse may also have protective functions for certain adults. Class distinction may be linked with concepts of abuse which suggest it is limited to a particular segment of society other than one's own, with the perception of abuse as limited to lower social classes being equally beneficial for middle class professionals and lay people. For example, there is substantial evidence that clients involved with social services in general and the child protection system in particular come from the lower socioeconomic classes (Gil 1970; Wolcock and Horowitz 1979; Pelton 1989; Creighton 1992). Recognizing that there is this social aspect to abuse would seem to suggest that a more equitable society would be the best way of minimizing abuse, however much intervention is oriented around individuals and families rather than at the structural level which requires large scale political and societal change.

From this it can be considered that while professionals possess discourses with common themes about child abuse and its management, these discourses must be seen in the context of adult, middle-class views of which they form a part, both influencing and being influenced by other definers such as the media, pressure groups and legislative bodies. Beliefs about child abuse are intimately bound up with beliefs about what is 'right' in society, and how society regards children and childhood; this is no less true for professionals than for lay adults. In this analysis, it can be considered that many professional views based upon the biopsychosocial understandings may be shared by lay adults, and that the tensions which are inherent in such a model can be utilized to support moral positions.

Whichever understanding of child abuse is dominant has direct and overt implications for the ways in which families are conceptualized and how we bring up our children. Within our culture, the family and the childrearing that is associated with it is a distinctly private matter. Embodied in this privacy is an implicit degree of secrecy and shared knowledge of family practices and culture that binds family members together. Thus, a family may be thought of as a number of people (adults and/or children) who share a common culture. Once exposed to public scrutiny the intricate bonds within the family may be severed, with family members feeling betrayed and unprotected. It is this deep-seated fear that creates so much concern regarding the definition of child abuse.

An analogy may be drawn between families and clothes. Families have several functions; for example, they provide mutual support to their members, just as clothes may have protective functions. In some situations, however, clothes are unnecessary and the wearing of them is culturally defined. For example, why do we wear swimming costumes when we visit our local swimming pool? We wear costumes because of complex cultural understandings about our genitals. Going swimming without a costume at a local pool would create a difficult situation for other swimmers and the pool attendants, who would probably not know how to react to such an unusual event. In the same way, the private parts of our families are hidden away from public gaze, despite family life being common to most of the population. The creation of family services allows us to acknowledge that families can and do have problems, and that solving problems may require input from outside the family unit. Solving family problems may reduce the incidence of child abuse. Thus conciliation services, which help to avoid or lead to a smooth divorce, may help to minimize the impact such adult actions have on the development of children.

There are few forums in which lay and professionals perspectives can be negotiated, but the child protection case conference is one such forum, and we will now develop a more detailed analysis of the involvement of lay views in this arena.

Lay views at the individual case level: case conferences

'Most of the research which has specifically addressed family involvement in child protection work has been concerned with *parents* at child protection *conferences*'. (Thoburn *et al.* 1995: 5) In relation to individual cases, the child protection case conference provides systematic coordination of professional intervention and has evolved a fundamental role in child protection procedures and practice (DHSS 1974; Hallett and Stevenson 1980; Hochstadt and Harwick 1985; British Association of Social Workers 1985). Conferences not only provide a focus for multidisciplinary coordination and decision making, but also have an informal agenda which includes maintaining inter-agency cooperation, sharing anxiety and protecting professionals (Moore 1985). Case conferences may also be extremely anxious situations, with professionals finding the atmosphere daunting and they are liable to rely on formal authority and ritualized professional behaviour (Hallett and Stevenson 1980). Moore (1985: 83) suggested that 'Workers are assembled . . . at a time of peak anxiety when a child has, or is thought to have been, abused . . .' and bring to the conference '. . . individual

feelings of denial, guilt, fear and anger'. It is in this forum that much professional consideration of lay views has been instituted through the involvement of families or, more specifically, parents in conferences.

The inclusion of parents in conferences has largely been practice-driven,
especially by social workers, who have a lead role in conference organization. While different professional groups may regard parental involvement
in different ways (Cooper and Pennington 1995), it is largely through social
work discourse that this issue has been considered (see, for example, Monk
1986; Corby 1987; McGloin and Turnbull 1987; Fallon 1992). This discourse is in accord with the prominence given to client self-determination
and ideas about partnership, which exist within contemporary social work
(Biehal and Sainsbury 1991).

This may be considered as very different from earlier notions of
professional–client relationships in child abuse management, when the ways
of understanding abuse were evolving from the biologically based medical
model. In the 1960s, for example, a major avenue for therapy was 'reparent-
ing', which was directed towards the maturation of the parents based on
such assumptions as some people were unable to control their own lives and
accept the responsibility for promoting change. The current ethos of including parents in decision-making meetings may therefore be considered as a
shift to the recognition that parents can accept responsibility for change,
and can be seen as a shift away from biological determinism to much more
of an emphasis on psychological and social influences.

Child protection differs from the many other areas where clients are involved, for example in mental health, because it is less easy to identify the
client. In the 1980s, public inquiries into child deaths frequently emphasized
that the child must be the prime focus of the case conference, and the Beckford and Spencer Reports (London Borough of Brent 1985; Derbyshire
County Council 1978) criticized social workers for making the family and not
the child the centre of attention. The Beckford Report stated that the principles of client self-determination that pervade social work are unsuitable in circumstances where abusing parents are attempting to care for children.

The inclusion of 'lay' people in conferences may be seen as an attempt to
incorporate lay views into the child protection arena. However, case conferences are difficult enough for professionals, and may not be the most
appropriate arena for allowing lay people to take responsibility. For example parents may feel intimidated by the professions. Farmer and Owen
(1995) described parents feeling threatened by the police presence in conferences as common, which emphasizes that child protection has legal as
well as health and social perspectives. Farmer and Owen also reported that
many parents in conferences appeared extremely anxious. In many ways,
the targeting of the case conference as the arena for the expression of
partnership with parents, allows the professionals to maintain rather than
devolve control of the case situation.

While literature and guidelines have suggested that the child is the main user of case conferences, those involved in child protection are required to consider the child in the family context, and this has been taken to include a consideration of the parents. These shifts in policies and practice in many ways reflect the difficulties in balancing the tensions between the rights of the parents and those of the child.

Unlike many other areas of social or health care, in which it may be considered beneficial to assimilate clients' views and understandings, within child protection there are strong policy and procedural guidelines for including parental views (Department of Health 1994), but at the same time equal and opposite forces regarding the rights of children mitigate against this. There is some evidence that by including parents in discussions, the views of children may be underrepresented (Taylor and Godfrey 1991). In Chapter 7, Nigel Watson argues that lay perspectives in health promotion allow for empowerment and challenge the dominant discourse in health. The inclusion of lay adult perspectives that challenge professional perceptions of a situation may be seen as verification that action is needed, because the individual or group expressing an alternative view may be considered by professionals to have failed to fully understand the situation. Christie (1993) illustrated this point when he considered how actions are interpreted in conferences: 'A difference in understanding emerged between professionals and carers about the nature of carers' questions. In general, carers said they asked "questions", whereas professionals described carers' questions as "challenges"' (p.195). This difference in perspective may be related to the involuntary nature of parents' 'participation'.

Diorio (1992) indicated that involuntary clients may have difficulties in negotiating professional input. Diorio (1992) demonstrated that many parents lacked an understanding of the roles and powers of statutory agencies. Parents often considered that agencies have much greater powers to make decisions and act against the family and child than they actually have. Diorio suggested that evaluation of service delivery from a parent's point of view has been largely avoided, as research has a traditional orientation around 'child saving', and there is also a lack of interest in the use of authority with involuntary clients. The casework method of practice prohibits client-based evaluation in its processes. The professional 'expert' may listen to the client, but then evaluate those views before translating them back to the client, thereby not working in partnership with the client's perceptions (Rhodes 1986).

Farmer (1993) suggested that there was a great discrepancy between social workers and parents on key issues in cases, such as who had abused the child, who was to blame and the degree of risk the child was currently facing. This disagreement increased difficulties in the working relationship. Farmer noted that such disagreement affected management in many ways, including the legitimacy of social work intervention. If the parents did not perceive that their child was at risk, they could see no reason for social work intervention.

Parents and professionals may therefore share a pool of potential understandings, but choose to utilize different levels of explanation of events to arrive at a more sympathetic or more accusing stance. For example, a mother suspected of hitting a two-year-old until she was bruised may stress the lack of social support she receives in caring for her children and the degree of stress she is under due to social conditions. The social worker may present a case that supports the mother in terms of her lack of support and difficult circumstances, thereby drawing upon social explanations. The doctor may emphasize the nature of the bruising and consider the degree of force necessary to produce it. The health visitor may present information regarding the physical development of the child and the quality of the mother–child relationship. Any information could be crucial in determining what the final explanation agreed by the professionals will be. The degree of force related to the bruising may indicate psychological help for the mother, whereas the health visitor's view that there is a good parent–child bond may endorse intervention based on social support. Once arrived at, the shared professional explanation is treated as 'correct', even when the family or an individual concerned favours an alternative explanation. The final professional explanation will therefore be arrived at through negotiation, and to some degree in a similar way to that suggested by Phil Barker and Chris Stevenson, on the basis of what resources are available.

The knowledge of the professional may be utilized to explain parental behaviour in the abuse investigation; therefore, the alternative view that challenges the professional view becomes evidence of 'hostility' or 'denial', which in turn shows that something is 'wrong' and that the professional explanation is right. Hostility to professionals in child protection may be conflict-specific and not characteristic of the individual involved. This hostility, however, may be inferred to be a parental trait based upon biology or psychology, leading to such 'treatments' as psychotherapy being directed at parents. When parents are uncooperative, children may be removed (Pelton 1989). For Diorio (1992), parental reactions to 'unjust' intervention by agencies may not be evidence of rationalization or resistance, but the response of a powerless party to a conflict situation. Frankel (1990: 50) recorded the attitude of one father to the conference as a 'load of old bollocks. You can't feed the kids on words'. This not only expresses dissatisfaction with the conference situation, but also implies that the father perceived his problems as financial to some degree.

When asked if parents' perceptions of a situation were important, especially in the acknowledgement of problems, one father said: 'If you're anti-authority, then you cannot have a discussion because they will just be blanking you out' (Frankel 1990: 51). This suggests it is not the parents' view that professionals do not respect, but the fact that the parent is challenging their dominant position.

Howitt (1992) noted that differences in professional and parental views do not prove anyone right or wrong, but instead indicate 'the way in which ideas about abuse are created within the context of professional activity' (p.5). This indicates that lay understandings at the individual case level are often difficult to reconcile with the professional conception of a situation, especially when the parental 'story' conflicts with professional attestation. Lay views are therefore accorded little legitimacy at the individual case level.

Shemmings and Thoburn (1990) asked parents about their ability to influence decisions. Some parents felt powerless: 'I didn't think my views carried any weight but they did listen to me. But our opinions carried no weight' (p.9). 'I felt they were all against me. Talking against me. They all backed each other up on everything they said. Oh yeah, but I feel parents should come' (p.10). This suggests that despite different professionals subscribing to different explanations of abuse, the amorphous nature of these explanations (as discussed in Chapter 5) allows one particular explanation to 'fit' a case and lead to appropriate intervention. It is also interesting to note that despite conferences often being dominated by social services professionals, the parents referred to all professionals as 'they'.

Christie (1993: 197), in reflecting on research undertaken in conferences commented: 'Although the focus of the research was on the experience of carers and professionals . . . we were surprised how seldom children were mentioned'. Christie's research may reflect the interaction that takes place within a conference, which is mainly in the domain of adults and largely excludes children. Although the case conference may be considered an adult forum in which children would have difficulty following and understanding what was going on (Morrison *et al.* 1990), children need information and want to hear what is being said about them (Taylor *et al.* 1993), and it may be considered that the case conference has evolved as it has because it has been developed from an adult perspective.

Taylor *et al.* (1993) evaluated children's views to investigation and protection in relation to sexual abuse. A year after disclosure, the children were asked who had been most helpful to them over this period; over 70 per cent reported either family members or friends, with almost half indicating their mother. Taylor *et al.* suggest that this implies that 'children place considerable reliance on the informal network in critical circumstances' (p.160). It also indicates that the potential loss of this network may prevent children seeking help. Despite the fact that most of the children were pleased they had reported the abuse, negative comments included: 'I didn't like the foster home. I was there for five months. The social worker told me it would only be five weeks. When I got taken away it was worse than the abuse' (ibid., p.162). This suggests that adults may see the stopping of abuse as reducing psychological stress, but the child in this case found the social circumstances more painful.

The implications of lay perspectives

By considering lay views in case conferences, it can be seen that the dominance of an explanation depends upon professional power, which leads one to suggest that lay people need to be empowered. Empowerment, however, is a problematic concept in itself. Sone (1993) indicated the complex process of attempting to support and empower parents, specifically non-abusing mothers. She described attempts to set up a self-help group and noted how some women were attracted to the counselling side of the service as a sanctuary, apart from the child protection issues rather than central to them. This indicates that clients may have needs that differ from professional perspectives of clients' needs. Sone also demonstrated the power inherent in empowerment: '*we* want a core of women who have been through the process to run a self help group' (Bernadette Manning, cited in Sone 1993: 17; our emphasis). This shows how user empowerment may be driven by the service provider, and may attempt to 'empower' people in a way that fits the professional child protection process, and allows it to move more smoothly rather than challenging it.

Empowering service users is not about empowering them to use the service, but to allow them to control their own circumstances and quality of life (Adams 1990). Acting in ways that give people power is not empowerment. Baistow (1994/95: 37) makes the following point:

> Those who do the empowering are increasingly likely to be health and welfare professionals . . . Those to whom empowerment is done are most likely to be users/clients/patients or employees. These are 'candidates' for empowerment because in professional estimations they need it doing to them or perhaps have a right to power.

Baistow considered that one view of empowerment suggests that the increasing 'colonization' of everyday life by professionals may involve empowerment that takes power out of the hands of professionals. For Baistow, this view tends to regard empowerment as independent of relationships, and she argued that rather than being disempowering to professionals, the empowerment process places professionals in a pivotal role. Professionals select suitable people to empower and this empowering role gives legitimacy to professionals and creates the 'expert role of empowerer' (Baistow 1994/95: 40). Making decisions about 'who should be empowered is a sign of power' (p.41). The empowerment of people becomes a professional task rather than a part of reflexive practice. Empowerment, therefore, has many of the tensions and contradictions found in child protection, and it does not necessarily challenge professional power and understandings, but may augment it.

So, for example, a mother who accepts that her partner has sexually abused her daughter and accepts professional views of what intervention is needed may be deemed a candidate for empowerment (Farmer and Owen

1995). A mother who denies the occurrence of suspected abuse is deemed to be uncooperative and not worthy of empowerment.

Lay views can provoke a more radical refocusing of the arena of child protection. Montgomery (1982) indicated that because child abuse is socially defined, it is dependent upon values rather than any objective judgement. Once society does define it and accepts that it occurs, it must do something to 'deal' with the 'problem'. With the acceptance of physical abuse (seen initially as psychopathological in origin), the medical profession was at the forefront of solving the problem. This they did by developing policies and procedures that identified children at risk and offering appropriate treatment to the abusing parents. This problem-oriented approach embraces narrow definitions that lead to interventionist strategies at a crisis level, rather than the broad conceptualization of child abuse such as that suggested by Gil (1979), which foregrounds more philosophical considerations. Again we can see that the formal explanation energizes the interventionist strategy.

La Fontaine (1990: 8) suggested that '. . . if children are to be protected, then the agency which protects them on behalf of society must have the power to intervene against any threat to them'. The protection of children is therefore synonymous with intervention (Howitt 1992) and not with prevention. Interventionist strategies control the family, and legislation that supports such intervention protects the state and child-protection workers from crisis and stress (Pfohl 1976; Parton 1985). We would also suggest that the interventionist strategy satisfies adult society's need for the management of abuse. When things 'go wrong' and there is a public outcry against too much/too little intervention, society has someone to 'blame' for the problem and official inquiries can identify the problems that need to be addressed so the system does not break down again.

An analogy can be drawn here between the medical model of disease and consequent intervention. If child abuse occurs, agents of the state must intervene, just as doctors must in the disease process. This focus on the 'disease' allows society to accept professional intervention and make it feel better, as it is getting something to alleviate the symptoms in much the same way as a prescription helps a patient. This disease perspective prevents a broader focus on preventative strategies. By defining the problem at an individual and family level, and focusing interventionist strategies at this level, adult middle-class society has created child abuse in which professional explanations are 'right', parental explanations either agree with professional views or are 'wrong', and explanations from the perspective of the child are largely ignored.

Conclusion

As suggested earlier, there is a developing discourse concerning the rights of children. This view of children in relation to child abuse and protection is, however, rather poorly understood. Explanations of abuse oriented around biological, psychological and social understandings drawn upon by adult professionals and lay people alike inhibit the broader philosophical stances that may be taken to child abuse. However, it is within these philosophical positions, as exemplified by Gil (1979), that the potential for an holistic approach to child abuse and child protection may lie. A better understanding of the child's perspective may help to transcend the tensions and conflicts inherent in the reductionist explanations which go to make up the biopsychosocial model.

7

Health promotion and lay health beliefs

Nigel Watson

Introduction

The aim of this chapter is to outline the place of lay health beliefs within the discourse of health promotion and to clarify the various models and frameworks within which lay beliefs are said to be important in encouraging changes in health experiences and behaviours. Health promotion is analysed in relation to biopsychosocial approaches and an analysis is made of the tensions that underlie the application of this model to changing health behaviours.

First, the concepts of health and health promotion will be considered. An overview of the literature on lay health beliefs will then be presented, and some of the key studies in this area will be used to demonstrate the potential importance of considering the views and beliefs of people when programmes intended to improve their health status are undertaken. It will be demonstrated that the social sciences have been the major contributor to the development of the literature on lay health beliefs, and the development of perspectives in this field will be outlined and areas of further development considered. By examining this literature, the potential challenge of lay health beliefs to professional models of health promotion will be demonstrated.

Health and health promotion

Health promotion is famously difficult to define. This can be attributed at least in part to the gap that exists between the ideal aspirations of its practitioners and the practical and political constraints of everyday life. However, it is also related to difficulties and disagreements about the concept of health. Clearly, if there is disagreement about the nature of health itself, then methods for its promotion are likely to be equally contentious.

For some authors, defining health is largely a philosophical process of concept clarification (Seedhouse 1986), whereas others take a more empirical approach and emphasize the differences in health status between social groups as a result of unequal access to health resources (Black Report 1980; Whitehead 1987). Beliefs and views about health also influence receptivity to changes in health behaviour and a discussion of lay health beliefs forms a central part of this chapter.

Health promotion involves a wide range of professionals, including doctors, nurses, road safety officers, teachers, environmental health officers, community workers and those who work in sport and leisure activities. Responsibility, though not usually authority, for the coordination of multidisciplinary initiatives normally lies with specialist health promotion officers working within the health service or local authorities. It is this second group of specialist, professionally qualified workers who are most likely to be involved in devising policies for the full range of health promotion activities, including the training of other professionals in the delivery of specific interventions.

Problems of definition are also closely linked to the breadth of activity and to the perceived need for intervention across societal and organizational levels and also by a range of different professional groups, all of whom will have their own professional cultures. It is common, for example, for doctors and nurses to encourage people to give up smoking at an individual level. However, health promotion practitioners argue that smoking as an individual activity is the outcome of a complicated process that also involves the needs of multinational companies (i.e. to make profits), advertising companies (i.e. to recruit new smokers) and governments (i.e. to raise large sums in taxation). Health promotion professionals often argue that in blaming the smoker we are blaming the victim (Naidoo 1986; Rodmell and Watt 1986). It is therefore commonplace for it to be argued that health promotion should include a wide range of preventative activities, including structural change as well as face-to-face education and advice. Locker (1991) reminds us that health promotion originates in a socioecological view of health, which places great emphasis on the links between individuals and their environment.

Jones follows a similar line of argument when she outlines the increasing emphasis on a social model of health that moves beyond disease or medical models, and which includes '. . . personal stories and lay accounts' as well as broader environmental issues such as income and housing and combines '. . . objective and subjective dimensions into a single framework' (Jones 1994: 543).

An emphasis on the wide range of health promoting activities, including individual behaviour change, community support for health, the creation of healthy environments and changes in national and global economic and fiscal policies, is generally important for an understanding of the ambitions of professional health promotion workers. It is particularly important for the purposes of this book, because of its resonance with the idea of a biopsychosocial model of health. Health promotion has always emphasized the need to tackle health issues by embracing a methodology that acknowledges that health is more than simply the absence of physical disease. As early as 1946, the World Health Organization defined health as '. . . a state of complete physical, mental and social well-being and not merely the absence of disease or infirmity'.

The definition was taken as an important legitimation for approaches to health promotion that challenged the biomedical model of health and its emphasis on disease pathology and the mechanistic treatment of physical disorder. It reflected the recognition that the prevention of illness is often more effective than its treatment and that the causes of disease are commonly attributable to social and environmental causes (McKeown 1976). This definition has been modified to encompass the notion of health improvement as an active and changing social process, as well as an attempt to achieve an absolute state of well-being (World Health Organization 1984).

Writing at around the same time, Ewels and Simnett (1985), both health promotion practitioners, emphasized the need to define health holistically and suggested that it should include 'a range of different dimensions classified as physical, mental, emotional, social, spiritual and societal' (pp.5–6). Despite continuing discussion and sometimes disagreement about methodology, this broad definition of health is still characteristic of most current health promotion activity and theory (Downie *et al.* 1990; Bunton and Macdonald 1992; Adams 1994). It is closely related to aspects of the new public health and often in conflict with the dominant discourse of biomedicine (Ashton and Seymour 1988).

There is a substantial literature which looks at the establishment of biomedicine as the current paradigm in medical practice (Foucault 1963/73; Jewson 1976; Armstrong 1983; Turner 1987; Stacey 1988) and, although it is not important to discuss this in detail here, it is necessary to suspend our unproblematic acceptance of scientific medicine as a neutral truth if we are to understand the importance of lay health beliefs within health promotion. Western medicine with its roots in the Cartesian separation of the mind and body has come to represent disease as an independent entity, or invader, which needs to be expelled. This is, of course, quite different from models of health and illness that emphasize the interdependent relationship between the individual and the environment. This latter idea is present in some alternative therapies, such as homeopathy, and also other medical systems, such as Chinese medicine (Stacey 1988; Aggleton 1990; Jones 1994).

However, the central issue for our purposes is to understand that bio-medicine is only one way, and not necessarily the right way, of establishing an explanation for ill health. It is sometimes difficult to stand far enough back from our own common sense understandings to accept that the power of scientific medicine is a matter of belief located in a number of assumptions about the objectivity of a specific approach to the body (Turner 1987). However, a number of commentators have pointed to the capacity in all cultures of healers to control the central definitions of health problems and most importantly the solutions to these problems. As Stainton Rogers states (1991: 18–19):

> From this perspective a combination of economic and professional dominance, and the threat posed by illness, enables healers *in all societies* not only to gain status and material advantage, and control access to resources, but also to promote their own explanatory systems . . . Their assumed superior skills, expert knowledge and high status provide them with the power to dispense healing or withhold it. Hence they gain the power to *construct* knowledge for others.
>
> (original emphasis)

This quote illustrates the core issues surrounding the place of lay health beliefs. Once normative discourse is made problematic, then the ideas of 'ordinary' people can be seen to have a different status and importance. Social constructionists argue that all illness is given its meaning through human and social definition. In this sense, disease cannot be properly understood aside from the context in which it is defined. For example, behaviours that in our culture will be classified as mental illness, will in other cultures be taken to indicate access to spiritual truth.

It should be clear by now that if we are to affect the way that people view their own health behaviour, then we need to start and take account of their beliefs and ideas and not discount these as subjective or as non-scientific.

Lay health beliefs and health promotion

Given the complex and wide range of approaches and topics that is encompassed within health promotion, it is not surprising that it has been influenced by a diversity of academic disciplines. The social sciences have been major contributors, although as Bunton and Macdonald (1992) demonstrate, the influences on practice and theory range more widely than this. Sociology, social anthropology and psychology have been the major contributors to the particular development of the literature on lay health beliefs.

Aggleton (1990) reminds us that ideas about, and definitions of, health vary considerably even within a particular society or culture, and the issues become more complex when we look at systems of medical practice other than Western biomedicine. Nevertheless, the process is not wholly a subjective one and consensus does exist about the nature and the value of what it is to be healthy. Aggleton makes a simple binary divide into 'official definitions and lay beliefs about health' (p.4), the former being the views of doctors and health professionals and the latter popular or non-professional views. Despite its simplicity, the division demonstrates a central issue: it underscores the debate regarding the control of the experience of health, especially in so far as language constructs that experience. It also exemplifies the tension and sometimes the divide between biomedical and social models of health. This is of critical importance for health promotion practitioners, because their core task is to act as an agent of change for health and, in particular, when this is directed towards the general population, the changes are only likely to be successful if they are congruent with the felt needs and beliefs of the recipients of the process of change. For example, there have been a number of educational campaigns regarding AIDS and HIV. While such campaigns have been considered effective in raising awareness (DHSS and Welsh Office 1987), there is little evidence that they have changed the behaviour of individuals. The beliefs held by an individual will affect his or her attention and response to campaigns, and lay beliefs will also be informed by other messages such as those in the media, which may present alternative and sometimes contradictory information to the public (Wellings 1988).

Morgan *et al.* (1985) argued that work in the field of health promotion has been characterized by two main approaches. The first of these has been to do with illness behaviour and originated in the concerns of the medical profession that patients were either not seeking help when they needed it or were not following advice when it was given. Clearly, this corresponds with Aggleton's official definition of health, in that it '. . . tended to accept providers' definitions of how the health service "ought" to be used and has generally sought to explain why these organisational solutions were not complied with' (Morgan *et al.* 1985: 76).

Morgan *et al.* go on to describe the second approach as rooted in a nominalist perspective in which no greater importance is attributed to medical knowledge than to lay knowledge. Such an approach is, of course, a challenge to the dominant medical model. The purpose of enquiry is '. . . to examine how the actor(s) interpret(s) and make(s) sense of disturbances in body functioning, with the decision to seek medical care being viewed as one possible response among a number of alternative courses of action.' (Morgan *et al.* 1985: 76).

While these ideas are positioned within a curative rather than a preventative framework, these differences are central to understanding the place of lay views in health promotion. Lupton (1994: 31) has argued that health education is '. . . a form of pedagogy which . . . serves to legitimise ideologies and social practices by making statements about how individuals should conduct their bodies', and although Lupton makes no attempt to distinguish between health promotion and health education, this is certainly true in terms of governmental initiatives such as the consultative document *The Health of the Nation*, which later became a White Paper (DoH 1992). This is not true, however, for those health promotion practitioners who are opposed to dominant ideologies on health, but instead are concerned with what they see as the essentially political nature of access to the means to achieve the desired health status at individual or community level. Rather than being centrally concerned with influencing the individual choice of lifestyle by individual consumers, health promotion should, they argue, be about advocacy for the disadvantaged and the redistribution of health resources in order to overcome inequalities and to achieve equity (Rodmell and Watt 1986). Participation is a central component in this process because it allows for the empowerment of those involved and because without it the dominant discourse cannot be challenged (Adams and Smithies 1990; Smithies and Adams 1993).

Health promotion is characterized by a range of complementary and sometimes competing perspectives on the best forms of practice and each of these is characterized by a different story about the relationship between practitioner and recipient (Beattie 1991, 1993). However, because of the commitment to change (at whatever level), with all of these perspectives a position has to be taken in relation to the views and beliefs of these recipients. These views range from the need of the public to change its health behaviour to conform with the instructions of the medical profession, to the medical profession being seen as a major barrier to the implementation of effective social health policies which require the empowerment of communities and a substantial redirection of resources towards those most in need. I hope that it is now clear that however these social, community and individual beliefs are taken into account, they nevertheless do need to be seen as central to health promotion programmes.

More detailed consideration of some of the key studies in this area demonstrate the potential importance of considering the views and beliefs of others when undertaking programmes for improving health status. As a formal process, this will apply irrespective of the value position of the practitioners involved, though the intended outcomes will vary. One of the earliest, but still much cited, examples of an alternative set of beliefs about health is Cecil Helman's (1978) study, 'Feed a cold, starve a fever'. As a GP who was also trained in social anthropology, he was especially well placed to study and report on the general beliefs that his patients held about disease causation and he used his findings to develop a 'folk model' of health. In reporting that his patients attributed key differences in terms of personal responsibility for colds and for fevers, he demonstrated that there were systematic and commonly held beliefs about the origins of everyday illnesses and that these could be shown to relate to common properties of 'cold' and 'hot' and of 'wet' and 'dry'. His subjects said that colds were caused by exposure to damp largely due to personal carelessness, whereas fevers were caused by germs that invaded the sufferer's body and so went beyond the control of – and therefore not the fault of – the individual.

Two points need to be made. First, is a basic example of how important it is to understand the belief system into which advice or information is placed. For example, if a health education campaign was aimed at encouraging individuals to take action to guard against some form of infection, it would be important to know that it was widely believed that this kind of illness was outside of individual control. Second, Helman attempted to establish the general and systematic nature of beliefs and he puts these forward as a model. Helman's work represents a good example of one way in which the study of lay health beliefs has been undertaken. However, other studies have been characterized by a concern with the particular and specific beliefs and practices of small-scale communities, and no assumptions have been made by their authors that a general model can be constructed. Some authors are concerned with the significance of the specific context, whereas others are more interested in general patterns. While there is no room here to explore the methodological and theoretical issues that follow from this difference, it is important to note the tension that exists between the attempt to establish regular patterns of human behaviour and the diversity and uniqueness of specific examples. In general terms, positivist studies will tend towards the establishment of general laws, while interpretative and social constructionist studies will tend towards a concern with specific context. It is also worth noting that it is well established that individuals are able to hold competing and contradictory beliefs about their health. We are able to recognize the contextual importance of explanations and to prioritize these in the light of the person to whom we are speaking. This ability is functional in avoiding conflict and in leaving open the range of individual behaviour options. It does, however, have significance if the purpose of a professional's encounter is to achieve behaviour change in another.

As already stated, the majority of studies that have addressed lay health beliefs have been concerned with commonsense ideas in relation to the causation of disease and illness within a curative context. Fewer studies have focused on a preventative or positive health framework. It is possible to apply the results of disease-related studies, though this relies upon the assumption that the subjects' beliefs can indeed be transferred from one context to another.

One researcher who has undertaken both types of study is Mildred Blaxter. Her early work was a small-scale ethnographic enquiry into the health beliefs of working-class mothers and daughters in Aberdeen (Blaxter and Paterson 1982). While much of this study was concerned with disease aetiology, the authors also looked into the sources of information that were valued by the different generations. This was done in an attempt to investigate the then much discussed idea of the cycle of deprivation. Their findings did not substantiate the normative view that the unhealthy lifestyles had occurred as a result of 'bad' habits being passed from generation to generation. Although grandmothers, mothers and daughters did share similar ideas about the broad nature of the concept of health and of the degree to which individual and personal control could be exercised against ill health, there were striking differences in the generational attitudes towards the health services. The younger women were much more likely to act as consumers and to be less deferential than previous generations. They were also less likely to accept advice and information from their mothers, relying instead on friends and expert health professionals. This has clear implications for the chosen methods of writing and sending health education messages.

However, we should always take care when considering the application of social scientific findings, because it is not unusual for there to be conflicting results in different contexts. From a social constructionist viewpoint, this is neither surprising nor a problem, since all social knowledge is considered to be contextual. For the practitioner, though, this can be confusing. Bloor and McIntosh (1990), for example, present an alternative perspective on the relationship between young mothers and the health visitor. Their research, which included an analysis of power relationships, emphasizes that their clients maintained control of the situation through various techniques of concealment and apparent agreement with the health visitor, while they were actually taking advice elsewhere and acting towards their children in ways other than those in line with the expert view. Perhaps the central issue is that for health education to be effective, it does need to take account of the specific contextual views and beliefs of the recipients, and these will need to be ascertained on each and every occasion through a process of active participation.

As mentioned above, Blaxter has also undertaken studies that have attempted to arrive at generalizations. The most recent of these was part of a very large-scale lifestyle survey (Blaxter 1990). While Blaxter's approach does not provide very much insight into beliefs or attitudes, her data do raise some surprising issues. For example, she found that in response to questions about the causes of disease, smokers were *more* likely to cite smoking as a factor and they also felt a greater degree of responsibility for their ill health than non-smokers. This indicates that attempts to discourage smoking need to incorporate help in stopping rather than information on smoking's harmful effects, which are already widely known. Another qualitative study (Backett 1992) also indicated that there is a complex interplay between an individual's knowledge of what they 'ought' to do and their capacity to implement these behaviours within the context of 'the social, moral and cultural constraints they experience in everyday life' (p.506). A related example is provided in a study of condom use by students (Middleton *et al.* 1994), which showed that despite knowing all the messages about safe sex, students stop using condoms because of the reduction in sensitivity and spontaneity. The implication is that this knowledge has to be addressed in health education, since it is not enough to assume that all individuals act in rational ways that deny their sensual experiences.

Blaxter (1990) also provides a classification of definitions of health. While older people are more likely to view health as a capacity to undertake functions in life, for example, Blaxter points out that for most people health is a multidimensional concept. A survey by Pierret (1993) in France resulted in the emergence of broadly similar lay definitions, though the survey was analysed in terms of discourse. There may be links with income, gender, occupation or age, but this is by no means a simple relationship; therefore, any effective health promotion programme needs to be sensitized to the perceived and felt needs of the client group.

Blaxter's overall conclusions in relation to health education are ambivalent. She remains convinced that socioeconomic and environmental factors have a greater impact on health than individual behaviours; she thus believes that educational programmes aimed at lifestyle change will not have a significant impact on their own 'because exposure to health risks is largely involuntary' (Blaxter 1990: 243). This would seem to indicate that the best programmes will be those which seek to work with the client group in the identification of those factors which arise from felt needs and which empower communities to tackle them collectively.

There has been considerable interest recently in developing a sociology of the body (Turner 1984, 1992; Martin 1987; Bordo 1990; Featherstone *et al.* 1991; Morgan and Scott 1993; Shilling 1993; Falk 1994), and there is also interest in trying to link concepts of the body and body image with health practices in general and health promotion in particular. Watson (1993) addressed the male body image and in so doing pointed to another neglected area of study, men's experience of health. He concluded that a narrow behaviourist focus on lifestyle is inadequate because it fails to pay attention to:

> the body's influence on male health experience, risks undermining the effectiveness of interventions designed to promote men's health . . . the issue is less one of communication and more a matter of addressing the 'missing' male body in the content of health education.
>
> (Watson 1993: 252)

Similarly, Saltonstall (1993) encouraged us to examine the experience of health, but went further in linking this to the situated construction of social order. In essence he argues that 'the interplay between health, self, body and gender at the individual level is linked to the creation and the recreation of a sense of healthiness in the social body, the body politic of society' (p.13).

Perhaps the issue here is in what way this linkage occurs. If the gaps between personal, community and expert discourse are wide, then one of the functions of effective health promotion should be to facilitate a flow between the levels. However, this should not mean the devaluing of lived experience in the face of expert denial, nor should it mean the failure to make explicit those inequalities in power relations that are structured by gender, ethnicity, class, sexuality or income.

Conclusion

I have attempted to illustrate that it is necessary for the social discourse and the practical activities of health promotion to be informed by the views of the public who are on the receiving end of the programmes. This is not at root a narrow matter of consumer consultation, but a more serious challenge to normative biomedical models and individualist ideologies. Williams and Popay (1994) remind us that the potential of this challenge is two-fold. Lay knowledge can both undermine the process of objectification that is the foundation for biomedical truth claims – it can be 'an epistemological challenge to expert knowledge' (p.120) – and it can also be a challenge to professional authority in the policy arena by presenting a 'political challenge to the institutional power of expert knowledge in general, and medical knowledge in particular' (p.120).

The issue of epistemological challenge is a central one within the overall framework of this book because issues of knowledge compatibility are at the core of any attempt to establish a biopsychosocial model of health. The main question then – and one that is much debated within the field of the philosophy of science – is whether the absolute claims of scientific knowledge can withstand the challenge of social constructionism. There is no need to discuss this in detail here except to say that superficial attractions of an holistic model of this kind may be masking basic tensions that will quickly emerge in practice once biological essentialism meets social relativism. The normative power of some truth claims and explanations – especially if they are backed up by government policy that is supported through a reliance on naive empiricism – means that the model is not a balanced one.

The political challenge may also be a contentious and unequal one. As stated earlier, health promotion as a practical process is undertaken by a very small number of specialists who rely on the cooperation and involvement of a wider range of professionals in the fields of health, welfare, education and the environment. In view of this, it could be argued that these groups are unlikely to be interested in lay health beliefs if these then lead to an undermining of their status and authority, and this remains a serious tension in any attempt to introduce a community-based health promotion project. Similarly, the repeated failure of governments to acknowledge the link between structural poverty and ill health, and instead to emphasize an individualistic model of personal responsibility, has left some of the most vulnerable in society with diminishing health and little voice in the process (Delamothe 1991).

There are clearly no simple solutions to issues such as these, which have their origins in much longer-standing debates about social justice and the truth of science. Perhaps, though, the central matter is a simpler one, in that power is inextricably linked to the capacity to be heard. If lay health beliefs can surface to more general levels of discourse, then perhaps greater democratization of the key processes may follow. Ulrich Beck (1992) has argued that in view of the environmental threats that now face us, it is not enough for science to be kept exclusively in the hands of scientists. As he states: 'The public sphere, in co-operation with a kind of public science, would be charged as the second centre of the discursive checking of scientific laboratory results in the crossfire of opinions' (p.119). Perhaps in a specific sense, this is the function of lay health beliefs within the discourse of medicine.

8

Cancer care: conventional, complementary or consensus

Shaun Kinghorn and Richard Gamlin

Cancer care: the challenge

In the UK, cancer is the second largest killer after heart and vascular disease. In 1991, more than 144,000 deaths were attributed to cancers, with some 206,000 new cases of cancer being diagnosed each year (George 1992). These statistics are alarming. Of further concern is the number of studies that have illustrated that cancer may be psychologically disruptive, (e.g. Greer and Moorey 1987; Cooper 1988). Pinnell (1988) goes as far as to suggest that cancer has become the scourge of the twentieth century.

The aims of this chapter are to appraise the relative merits of biomedical and complementary therapies within the management and prevention of cancer; to explore the tensions that exist between medicine and complementary therapies from research, organizational and practice perspectives; and to consider the scope for reconciling the two types of therapies.

Confusion exists in the media, in society and in medicine about the aims of cancer care. Broadly speaking, the debate is between curative and palliative care. Faithfull (1994) suggests that, for the patient, cure is perceived not only as the absence of disease but also the resumption of life prior to having cancer. In contrast, medicine often perceives cure as disease-free survival. Palliative care, is defined in the context of this chapter as the total care of patients whose disease is not responsive to curative treatment. Control of pain, of other symptoms and of psychological, social and spiritual problems is paramount. The goal of palliative care is achievement of the best possible quality of life for the patients and their families.

Biomedicine and conventional treatment

For most of this century, surgery, radiotherapy and chemotherapy have provided the mainstay of approaches to treating cancer, both curatively and palliatively. In a 1992 US survey, Weiss (1993) noted that one million new cases of cancer were diagnosed, half of whom died. With cure rates for all cancers standing at approximately 50 per cent, there has not been a significant reduction in total mortality rates over the last fifty years. Regarding chemotherapy, Priestman (1989) noted that it has become increasingly clear that much of the promise offered by drug treatment during the 1960s and 1970s has not been fulfilled. Furthermore, Weiss (1993) has stated that since the passing of the National Cancer Act under the Nixon Administration, few curative discoveries have been made.

Webb (1988) noted that advances in treating cancer have increased the chances of finding a cure. Such cautious optimism is not shared by Stoll (1991), who implied that the positive impact on cancer treatments is an illusion constructed by popular media in the USA and Europe. Such an assertion is supported by Brewin (1994) citing Robin Day, who in his memoirs wrote of television's inherent tendency to distort.

Despite earlier diagnosis and more effective treatment, the overall incidence of cancer in the UK has risen by 10 per cent (Laurance 1994). In some respects, health care disciplines demonstrate a certain degree of naivety when comparing the impact of medicine on cancer mortality and morbidity rates. Medicine has made significant in-roads in improving the chance of life as well as the quality of life. Drugs such as interferon and tamoxifen and therapies such as stem cell harvesting may alter significantly the prognosis of the cancer patient and much hope has been invested in genetic manipulation. But the belief that medicine will, by itself, conquer cancer is an illusion.

Unguarded optimism is premature if we are to learn from the unbridled enthusiasm associated with the development of cytotoxic therapies. The well-documented evidence of cancer cure statistics has, to a certain extent, been overshadowed by the impact of cancer treatments on the individual's quality of life. The cure is often perceived to be worse than the disease itself. Cancer treatments are unique in terms of their likely impact. Green and Kinghorn (1994) pointed out that in the eyes of some patients, radiotherapy is synonymous with a death sentence. Decker *et al.* (1992) also suggested that cancer treatment often causes stress, anxiety and depression. Eardley (1986) examined patients' attitudes and knowledge towards radiotherapy and found that 43 per cent of those involved in the study believed the treatment to be painful. It is this increasing awareness that orthodox medicine has limits so far as cure and promoting comfort is concerned, which has led to a greater emphasis being placed on complementary therapies as a configuration of approaches that can provide more acceptable forms of treatment.

Complementary therapies: what do they have to offer?

It is difficult to find a clear definition of complementary therapies. Fulder (1988) defines complementary therapies as those therapies which are not covered by the traditional undergraduate medical curriculum. In contrast, Lewith (1993), citing the British Medical Association, suggested that non-conventional medicine can be defined as those forms of treatment which are not widely available and used by orthodox health care professionals. Neither definition is particularly useful because they fail to capture the breadth and relevance of complementary therapies in cancer care.

Complementary therapies are often described as natural, safe, holistic, gentle and harmonious. Some – for example, traditional Chinese medicine and acupuncture – have been practised for centuries. It is reasonable to assume that complementary therapists offer time, privacy and individual attention within the promised holistic approach. Patients feel the need to approach complementary therapists because they are unable to get this sort of attention from conventional health care.

The demand for complementary therapies usually originates in and from the community, whereas access to conventional cancer care is controlled by the professional. The emergence and growth of complementary therapies is sustained by an overwhelming desire to offer a counter-culture against a discipline which has removed the fundamental right of the community to influence.

In the same way that death has been taken over by the funeral director, cancer care is principally the domain of medicine, which, as a discipline, embraces epidemiology, treatment and cure, and mortality as its fundamental principles. The result is that cancer care has become 'tumourcentric' at the expense of perspectives on the social, emotional and spiritual dimensions of life. For many, complementary therapies may be perceived as a source of hope when the medical prognosis is that nothing more can be done. Complementary therapies also allow individuals to gain some control over the management of their cancer. For example, a number of therapies require self-referral. As a result, the person decides who delivers the therapy and when. In conventional cancer treatments, the oncologist is the main orchestrator of the nature and timing of treatments.

Buckman and Sabbagh (1993) offered a sensitive and conciliatory critique of complementary approaches to health care. They asked whether orthodox and/or complementary therapies are 'Medicine or Magic'? and concluded that all therapy contains an element of both: 'Diseases need medicine, but human beings will always need a touch of magic' (p.235).

Getting better or feeling better?

When considering cancer care it is important to consider morbidity as well as mortality. Many of the arguments and counter-arguments between complementary and conventional carers revolve around these issues. The conventionalists claim that complementary therapists may help the patient to feel better, but do nothing to arrest the disease process, while complementary therapists claim that much of conventional cancer care is based on cutting, poisoning and burning. This debate was most noticeable in the research carried out by Bagenal *et al.* (1990) at the Bristol Cancer Help Centre to examine the effects of complementary therapies on breast cancer. As Lloyd (1992) noted, the headlines following the publication of the study indicated that women with breast cancer who had attended the Centre were three times more likely to suffer a relapse. It later emerged that the study was flawed because of lack of comparability between the study and control groups. Yet, to date, there appears to be no firm evidence that complementary therapies can be considered to be a major curative intervention.

It is often assumed that little or no research is available to support the assertion that complementary therapies have a knowledge base that legitimizes their acceptance and use. However, there are many examples of research that can, at least, inform practice. Yearwood-Dance (1992) found relaxation reduced symptom distress in patients receiving radiotherapy. Scott *et al.* (1986) conducted a comparative trial of clinical relaxation and an anti-emetic drug regime and found that the total emetic period was four hours shorter in the relaxation group, although the intensity of vomiting was greater in this group.

There is a pervasive belief among health practitioners that the person seeking complementary therapies does so as a last resort. Yet according to Fiore (1979) and Cassileth (1982), patients are generally well educated, frequently asymptomatic at the time of their first consultation with a complementary therapist and in the early stage of their disease. This is not without its problems, as patients may be misinformed that the complementary therapy being offered is curative rather than palliative. Downie *et al.* (1994) noted in a piece of research to investigate the usage of complementary therapies in oncology units, that patients perceived complementary therapies as offering more hope than conventional approaches. For a small group of patients, cure was cited as the reason for receiving complementary therapies. In terms of survival, the patient may be better off receiving orthodox therapies. Experience informs us that, in a small number of cases, people abuse their position as practitioners by being conservative with the truth about their therapeutic approach.

From the preceding arguments, it can be seen that both conventional and complementary treatment approaches to caring for patients with cancer have much to offer patients and their carers. However, tensions exist between the two approaches.

Complementary therapies and conventional cancer care: tensions and resolutions

Medicine has a rich and long history of supporting the validity of its therapies via systematic scientific inquiry. There is extensive clinical research into the aetiology, prevention, treatment and management of cancer with some clinical journals devoted exclusively to cancer. Organizations such as the Imperial Cancer Research Fund, the Cancer Research Campaign and Marie Curie Cancer Care devote time, expertise and considerable amounts of money to cancer research.

It is inevitable that the anecdotal knowledge base of some complementary therapies has become a major source of concern for those engaged in conventional cancer treatments. Gaining acceptance, rather than ridicule, by the medical profession, presents complementary therapists with a major challenge.

A scientific base for cancer care

Despite a long history of inquiry, developing a scientific basis to cancer care is itself problematic. Most would agree that sound scientific research should be the foundation of all interventions, but research is costly both in time, skills and resources. The subjectivist foundation of complementary therapies is perhaps the greatest stumbling block to medicine and alternative approaches to cancer care being equally valued. Andrew Vickers, research officer at the Research Council for Complementary Medicine, speaking at the Second National Staff Nurses' Conference, criticized nurses for using a wide range of complementary therapies that have not been evaluated. His position was that research on the most popular therapies such as aromatherapy, massage and reflexology has been inadequate. The *Nursing Times* receives many papers from nurses who cite references as providing evidence for the use of a complementary therapy. However, when refereed, a large number of the papers turned out to be introductory guidebooks offering no research to support the therapeutic claims they make (*Health Visitor* 1994). If complementary therapies are to be used safely and effectively and taken seriously, it is not only essential for therapists to engage in research but to make use of published material. Lewith (1993) cites a document by the British Medical Association entitled 'Complementary medicine: New approaches to good practice', which while recognizing that randomized controlled trials are not the only method of evaluating therapies, suggested that complementary therapies must utilize existing research methods used within conventional medicine.

The lack of a research base has led to complementary therapies being described as unscientific (Laffan 1993). The effectiveness of complementary approaches as curative interventions is open to conjecture; therefore, it would be unethical to sanction studies into the effectiveness of complementary remedies without a rational basis. Patients are often willing to participate in conventional anti-cancer drug trials in the hope of a cure. But what rationale can be given for a clinical trial using a complementary approach? However, we will remain ignorant of the curative or supportive potential of complementary therapies if they are not taken forward in rigorous clinical trials. An example of a specific therapy illustrates the advantages of scientific, research-based evaluation.

Aromatherapy is currently enjoying great popularity. The popular press regularly publishes articles extolling the virtues of massage with essential oils, and the general public could be forgiven for believing that aromatherapy is the cure for all ills. It may well have something to offer beyond the widely accepted view that pleasant smells can make one feel better. Wilkinson (1995) investigated the effectiveness of aromatherapy massage in enhancing the quality of life for patients receiving palliative cancer care. Although it is beyond the scope of this chapter to offer a comprehensive review of this research, it became evident that aromatherapy massage may have a significant role in enhancing the quality of life for cancer patients. Perhaps one of the most interesting features of this study was its use of established research tools such as the Rotterdam Symptom Checklist (De Haes *et al.* 1990) and the State Anxiety Inventory (Spielberger *et al.* 1983). The use of such recognized tools, combined with randomization of the sample, suggests that critiques levelled at complementary therapies being unproven is premature and without substance.

Much conventional medical research begins with controlled clinical trials on healthy volunteers. It would seem that aromatherapists could begin their journey into scientific research in a similar way, as illustrated by Wilkinson (1995). For example, it would be relatively easy to measure various physiological parameters before and after the introduction of a single or combination of essential oils. A range of psychological tests and quality of life scores exists that might usefully be employed in such clinical trials. Although trials with healthy volunteers will not provide the data required to decide whether or not aromatherapy is effective in cancer care, they may provide a way for therapists to be taken seriously by the scientific community.

As stated above, orthodox therapy relies on scientific methods that rigorously dissect, evaluate and strive to correct disease as a basic molecular process. Complementary literature is, in the main, based on anecdote and subjective responses (Burk and Sikora 1992). Complementary therapies are, allegedly, based upon witchcraft and mystery, and devoid of scientific rigour. It is the differing perspectives on the validity of therapies and the attendant knowledge bases that provide perhaps the greatest tensions. West (1992) pessimistically suggested that medical and scientific journals deride alternative medicine as the flight from science. Medicine, arguably, sees itself as the guardian angel of therapeutic intervention and scientific rigour provides the entry gate to quality patient care. Weil (1983) believes that doctors invite patients to dream along with them, that the clear light of medical science will erase all superstitions of the past, including all rival systems of treatment and with them the diseases that plague humanity – even, perhaps, death itself. They want everyone to see them as real scientists and medicine as real science. Other disciplines allied to medicine may owe their professional standing to being research-based in a similar vein to medicine.

One can understand the anxiety of the protagonists of the medical model in view of the threat that complementary therapies offer to the dominance of medicine in the management of cancer. Since knowledge is often described as having latent or implicit power, medicine is sometimes quick to draw on its empirical armoury in discrediting research into complementary therapies in a prejudicial manner. However, conciliatory and restrained commentary is essential if these two models of care are to be successfully integrated. Cancer and cancer treatment has a history, a politics, a mainstream and a lunatic fringe (Kabat-Zinn 1994). One has to remember that modern chemotherapy owes its conception to the serendipitous observation that mustard, used as an agent of war, was also potent in the 'war' against cancer. Polarizing the bases of conventional and complementary approaches is neither helpful, truthful or productive in reconciling the differences between the two perspectives. In terms of the respective knowledge bases, where do the tensions lie?

In response to the scientific medical approach to cancer care, complementary therapists may argue that their therapy is not amenable to the standard double-blind, crossover trial. Medicine itself is not immune from such research dilemmas. McWhinney *et al.* (1994) pointed out that randomized trials may prove impracticable when trying to evaluate palliative care services scientifically. Scarcity of subjects is a problem faced by researchers in both complementary and conventional cancer care. The single-case experiment (Hersen and Barlow 1976) is one way of overcoming this difficulty. Single-case experiments measure change in individuals over a period of time during which various treatment options are introduced in a controlled manner. The approach has been adopted in psychology (Yule and Hemsley 1977) and also in nursing (McLeod *et al.* 1986; Guyatt *et al.* 1988; Newell 1992). Alternative inquiry positions are the case-study approach and 'softer' qualitative research methodology.

Reason and Rowan (1981) and Lincoln and Guba (1985) present a radically different and perhaps opposing view of 'science' known as 'new paradigm' research, or cooperative experiential inquiry. They question the validity of manipulating variables where human beings are concerned and warn against projecting the results of laboratory studies onto the real world. The goal of new paradigm research is to gain information and knowledge that is useful to all who participate in the study. It is not suggested that orthodox approaches to scientific research should be abandoned, but that new paradigm research may have much to offer when studying people. New paradigm research methods should be no less rigorous than orthodox methods. New paradigm research has much to offer in the field of complementary therapies in cancer care and treatment; however, it is not an alternative to scientific inquiry, which still offers the greatest hope in finding 'a cure for cancer', or to developments in treatment and management.

Examples of relevant new paradigm research include the study by Reason (1988), which was based upon a cooperative inquiry group that was set up to explore the theory and practice of holistic medicine. Following an introductory planning meeting, the cooperative inquiry group met for a two-day workshop. The co-researchers spent six weeks in practice and concluded their study with a four-day workshop. The study enabled doctors to review their own practice in the light of their colleagues' practice, and to explore new ways of caring for others. Throughout the study, the participants were treated as equals. 'Data' were not taken away for processing by the primary researcher, but constantly fed back to the group in an action–reflection–action cycle. The approach was consistent with the aims of the study and attempts at reducing alienation. It honours participants as human beings with a free will and self-determination. In common with other cooperative inquiries, this study was intense and time-consuming and therefore expensive, but these constraints were outweighed by the direct benefit to the participants who were immediately able to influence their practice.

Organizational issues/practice issues: meeting the demand for complementary therapies

In the light of current health care reforms, patients are being invited to tell health care planners and providers what they want from their care service (Speechley 1992; Spiers 1994). In the Cancerlink document, 'A declaration of rights for people with cancer', it is stated that people have a right to a second medical opinion, to reject treatment or to undertake complementary therapy without discrimination to continued medical services. We can infer from this that demand for complementary therapies for people with cancer is likely to increase. With European legislation stating that within the next ten years the NHS should be providing complementary therapies, we are likely to witness a burgeoning of these services, especially for patients with cancer (Tattam 1992). In a survey of uptake of complementary therapies across Europe from 1985 to 1992, Fisher and Ward (1994) note that 26 per cent of people in the UK reported having used a complementary therapy. Although it was acknowledged that there were some methodological flaws in collating the figures, the study indicated that a significant proportion of the population are using non-conventional approaches. Are those who are currently planning future health care provision in touch with present and future demand for alternative therapies? In an article in the *British Medical Journal* entitled 'The future of medicine', Morrison and Smith (1994) make no overt reference to the potential for incorporating complementary therapies into medicine. This is not a healthy position to take in view of anticipated demands for these alternative approaches.

Delivering complementary therapies

If complementary therapies have no immediate appeal or relevance to medicine, who is going to provide these therapies to cancer patients? Denton (1992) claims that people we care for are demanding that nurses should be in a position to offer a wide range of therapeutic skills. The principle of advocacy suggests that patient empowerment, control and choice are fundamental. Flaherty (1981: 40) stated that: 'There are options we can explore, approaches we can try and steps we can take to help ourselves . . . please give us the power and sense of control'. But if nursing is to thrive in the complementary therapy arena, it needs to adopt scientific rigour. Fitch (1992) suggested that oncology nursing research began because there was a desire for good information to make reliable and valid clinical decisions regarding the care of individuals with cancer and their families. In reality, are nurses in a position to absorb another sphere of practice into their repertoire of skills? Will Trusts and GP fundholders support study leave and refund the expenses incurred to ensure practitioner competency?

Since quality cancer care is multidisciplinary in nature, it would seem inappropriate for one specialist group to monopolize the delivery of complementary therapies. Indeed, many practitioners such as clinical psychologists and occupational therapists already have established programmes that prepare them for using certain approaches, such as relaxation techniques and mental imagery. It would therefore appear expedient for managers of services to develop an inventory of which disciplines are already prepared and in a position to offer a particular facet of complementary therapy. The expansion of complementary therapies based on provision via a variety of disciplines is likely to diminish the risk of any one discipline monopolizing this important range of therapies.

Safety and quality

Over the last five years, the drive to articulate quality of care has gained considerable momentum. Many of the current approaches to treating cancer such as chemotherapy have undergone rigorous trials. Their delivery is often based on clearly defined protocols, with practitioners having undergone specialist training. Conversely, the majority of complementary approaches have yet to offer firm, clear guidelines for delivering a therapy, even though complementary therapists may have undergone a form of specialist training. This fact, combined with the small number of regulatory/disciplinary bodies for a wide range of diverse therapies, will not appeal to NHS Trusts. A situation has arisen where purchasing complementary therapies is an area of uncertainty.

How does a particular unit or individual recognize when an alternative therapy has been delivered in a safe and effective manner? If the therapy has been harmful, who does the patient with cancer turn to? Presently, physiotherapists, nurses and doctors are governed by regulatory bodies. Corresponding bodies in the areas of complementary therapy are sparse and embryonic in their development. Fisher and Adam (1994) note there are currently five bodies regulating complementary therapies in the UK. It is blatantly obvious that the majority of different therapies are not represented in these five bodies. So far as nursing is concerned, the Code of Professional Conduct (UKCC 1992) considers that nurses should always act to promote and safeguard the interests and well-being of patients, acknowledge any inadequacies in their knowledge and competence, and desist from undertaking any duties that cannot be undertaken in a safe and competent manner. This poses a number of dilemmas. The person with cancer may request the administration of a substance that is unproven. Is the nurse therefore acting in the best interests of the patient if he or she obliges? Yet according to the declaration of rights, patients ought not to be viewed in a prejudicial manner if they wish to go along the complementary therapy route. Every provider of cancer care will have to put policies in place to guide practitioners in the management of these dilemmas.

On this theme, Lewith (1993) noted that when a doctor refers to a nonmedically qualified therapist, he or she still retains legal responsibility for diagnosis and management of the patient. One can understand the reluctance of conventional medicine to engage the services of an alternative practitioner whose preparation for practice is not validated by research and/or codes of practice. This degree of uncertainty has created a situation where the threat of litigation may impede the rapid development of complementary therapies in centres of cancer care. Although individual practitioner insurance may ease this threat, the awareness that bad publicity linked with the use of unproven approaches may threaten the prestige of large cancer centres.

If one is to consult any practitioner for cancer care, one has the right to assume that the practitioner will be competent. If one consults a doctor, nurse or other conventional practitioner, one can assume with reasonable confidence that he or she is competent to practice. In the case of complementary therapists, it is much more difficult to ascertain their competence. As was noted above, it is clear that the doctor who refers a patient to a non-medically qualified therapist still retains legal responsibilities for diagnosis and subsequent management. One tension that has arisen surrounding this issue has emerged from the use of massage for patients with cancer. Oldfield (1992) notes that massage has been shown to stimulate the lymphatic system. In the case of breast cancer, the lymphatic system has clearly been identified as a pathway by which the tumour may spread. In breast cancer, the use of arm and shoulder massage may in fact accelerate the spread of the tumour via stimulation of the lymphatic system. This example illustrates the real tension that exists when complementary therapies and conventional approaches are used conjointly.

The problem is compounded when the doctor is unaware that the patient is undergoing complementary therapy, because the patient does not choose, or is afraid, to discuss the matter with the doctor. Serious reservations are expressed by orthodox practitioners who share the care of their patients with non-medically qualified complementary therapists. A similar tension is found in diagnosis. Iridology and reflexology are examples of complementary therapies where diagnosis is a major feature of the therapeutic package. Since diagnosis historically has been the domain of medicine when such therapies engage in diagnosis, tension between conventional and complementary therapies arises. Complementary diagnosis is intrusive to conventional professional boundaries. Staff providing traditional cancer care often have a wide range of qualifications up to degree level and beyond. This is not to suggest that all complementary therapists must hold a degree in medicine and surgery, but that a working knowledge of the human body and the principles of cancer care would seem fundamental for patient comfort and safety.

Conclusion

It is often perceived that medicine and complementary therapies hold the key to *dealing with* cancer in terms of cure and promoting comfort. Such a premise is illusory. Yet Doll and Peto (1981) suggests that in theory 80 per cent of all cancers are preventable. Both medicine and alternative approaches do not focus essentially on prevention. Both are clamouring for the high ground of cure or comfort and its associated prestige. Both approaches catch the cancer patient as he or she falls under the 'shadow of the crab'.

One obstacle to the acceptance of complementary therapies has been claims for curing cancer via complementary measures. The consequent, fruitless debate has eroded the true value of complementary therapies in providing comfort. When used in combination, complementary and conventional therapies can be a major force in enhancing the quality of life of cancer patients and their families during all phases of the cancer experience.

Decker *et al.* (1992) found that relaxation therapy for those receiving radiotherapy brought about reductions in tension, depression and anger. A collaborative cancer care initiative between Hammersmith Hospital and the Bristol Cancer Centre reassures us that both orthodox and alternative therapies can co-exist for the benefit of cancer patients and their families.

Complementary therapies are starting to develop an empirically based body of knowledge, but this progress has yet to be acknowledged by orthodox medicine. If the desirable combined therapeutic approach is to emerge, then medicine needs to respect complementary approaches. In a letter in the *British Medical Journal*, Vickers (1994) suggested that doctors should routinely ask patients about their usage of complementary therapies while taking an admission history. Since the majority of complementary therapists practise outside a NHS provider setting, such information will help patients recognize that medicine acknowledges that the need for hope and comfort is not comprehensively dealt with by orthodox cancer treatments.

Conventional medicine is governed by the principles of audit, standards, protocols and other forms of regulations, which if embraced by complementary therapists might bring about more conciliatory dialogue. This in turn may protect patients with cancer who are looking for therapeutic approaches that offer, in whatever shape or form, comfort, cure and hope. Perhaps the greatest progress would be made if these two perspectives were to develop shared goals. Conventional medicine has an extensive research knowledge base reducing cancer treatment and cure. In return, medicine would be greatly enhanced by its contact with complementary therapies through a focus on a more holistic and less mechanistic view of people with cancer. People need medicine and magic.

9

The social construction of grief

Glynis Hale

The activity of constructing and/or generating models of human experience is very much a product of twentieth-century biosocial sciences (Henriques *et al.* 1984), and the bereavement experience has not escaped this modelling culture. Concepts such as 'the grief reaction' (e.g. Lindemann 1944; Parkes 1972; Rabin and Pate 1981; Worden 1983; Youngson 1989) and 'the grief process' (e.g. Bowlby 1961, 1980; Gorer 1965; Hoagland 1983; Stroebe *et al.* 1993) can be seen as the culmination of over 50 years research into bereavement experiences. While many practitioners argue that such models are used merely to provide guidelines for working with bereaved individuals, my experience both as client and as counsellor suggests that they are frequently used in a prescriptive rather than reflexive way. The aim of this chapter is to address some of the issues raised by existing models of grief, specifically issues around the appropriateness of the models themselves and the potential implications of their imposition onto individual experiences of grief. It will be suggested that these issues (together with the consequent theoretical and practical tensions) are grounded in the pervasive adoption of a biopsychosocial model of grief by both the researcher and practitioner working within this field. I will argue that such a model, while claiming to be 'holistic' in the sense of adopting a multidimensional explanatory framework, is firmly located within an essentialist model of the person, which constrains – even directs – the nature of research and practice in this area. Thus, the issues and tensions arise as a consequence of working from a model of human experience that is inappropriate and unsustainable when viewed in the context of the bereavement experience.

First, let me provide a brief overview of the literature of bereavement. The earliest systematic study of this area is conventionally credited to Linde-mann (1944) and his work with individuals bereaved under a variety of circumstances. The results of his interviews suggested a 'typical' response to bereavement, which included somatic symptoms, preoccupation with the dead person, anger and guilt, behavioural changes and psychosomatic ill-ness. Although Lindemann's methodology and subject sample have since been criticized (see, for example, Parkes 1972; Lofland 1985; Middleton *et al.* 1993), this work served to open up a new area of human experience to interdisciplinary enquiry. Since then, there have been thousands of studies directed towards a clearer elucidation of bereavement experiences, and it would be impossible to do justice to the scope and complexity of such studies here. However, the general aim of these studies has been to identify factors influential in the nature and development of grief, and to clarify the significance of these factors so as to identify those most 'at-risk' of de-veloping 'complications' in their response to bereavement.

The current position is one which attempts to integrate understandings of bereavement into some form of multidimensional model, a model that re-cognizes the role of the many different influences on grief. For example, Shuchter and Zisook (1993) propose six dimensions that must be acknowl-edged and addressed in the individual's experience of bereavement. The relationship between these dimensions has yet to be determined, but this particular approach seems to be viewed as 'the way forward' in increasing our understanding of bereavement experiences. However, even as meth-odological rigour increases and understandings become more complex, con-cern has frequently been expressed as to the plausibility and utility of grief research to date. Kamerman (1988: 68–9) urges caution when he comments that, 'taken together, it is clear that grief follows patterns, although the room for individual variation is considerable'.

To what extent can the complexity of a multidimensional approach allow space for such variation to emerge? Cochran and Claspell (1987: 30) ex-press this concern even more strongly when they argue that, 'no list of symptoms rises above a rather disorderly collection . . . [and] . . . whatever unity emerges is imposed from our prior knowledge of what grief is'. Thus there is a tension between the continuing development of increasingly soph-isticated models of grief and a perception that such developments serve to constrain what is in reality an extremely complex experience. But what is the source of this tension? How and why has it occurred?

It is suggested here that the basis of this tension can be found in the pervasive adoption of an essentialist, biopsychosocial model as the 'meta-theory' within which the majority of bereavement research is, and always has been, undertaken. This essentialist approach rests on the assumption that human behaviour and experience is the ultimate manifestation of uni-versal inner states or 'essences'. Diversity in the expression of these essences is seen to reflect the influence of a wide range of individual and social factors impinging on the person at any given time (see Eisenbruch 1984). Hence, this approach distinguishes between 'grief' as an inner state and 'the grief reaction' as the outward manifestation of that state following its mediation by personal and social factors.

However, Harré (1986: 4) argues that such a view is based on incorrect assumptions about the nature of 'emotions':

> Psychologists have always had to struggle against a persistent illusion that in such studies as those of emotion there is something *there*, the emotion, of which the emotion word is a mere manifestation. This ontological illusion, that there is an abstract and detachable 'it' upon which research can be directed probably lies behind the defectiveness of much emotion research. In many cases the only 'it' is some physiological state which is the basis of some felt perturbation. Swayed by the ontological illusion, it is easy to slip into thinking that that state is the emotion.

I would argue that it is this 'illusion' of an inner state of essential 'griefness' which has directed the course of grief research to date. In so doing, this inner state has been ascribed primacy over all other influences; that is, the assumption that without an essential 'grief' there would be no 'grief reaction'. In reality, the opposing story is equally plausible; that is, that there would be no concept of 'grief' without the sociocultural context which constructs and defines it as such. This is not to suggest that there would be no 'sympathetic nervous system perturbation' without a sociocultural context, but that such perturbation *in itself* cannot constitute 'grief' or the 'grief reaction'.

The methodological limitations of this model of grief have already been highlighted in the preceding discussion, focusing as it does on the complexity of bereavement experiences and the emergent tensions within the literature of this area. However, this is but one area of concern; the adoption of a biopsychosocial model has further consequences for our understanding (or misunderstanding) of bereavement experiences at both the theoretical and the practical level of operation.

On a theoretical level, the location of grief research within the constraints of a biopsychosocial framework has created a need for explanation and justification of variations on the course of the grief process and the nature of the experience itself. Diversity must be accounted for, primarily by reducing experience to the biological, the psychological and/or the social. As Parkes (1972) comments 'each of [the] stages of grieving has its own characteristics and there are considerable differences from one person to another as regards both the duration and the form of each stage' (Parkes 1972: 27).

On the basis of this statement, one could imagine the extreme scenario in which, initially, the bereaved person will appear to be shocked or numbed by the death, or then again they might not. Next comes the stage at which they will deny that the death has really occurred, or then again they might not, or they may even pass through this stage first. Next comes the stage of 'real grief', which is itself impossible to define and which can include almost any experience one can imagine. However, one must not assume that this stage will come next; it may be experienced immediately after the bereavement, or the bereaved person may revert from anger and denial back to appearing numb and shocked, always assuming they have passed through these stages previously. If they have not, then stages 1 and 2 (based on existing biopsychosocial models) become stages 2 and 3 when they are finally experienced after the stage of 'real grief'. Finally, there is a stage of acceptance and reorganization. But even at this point it is still possible to revert to an earlier stage, whatever that stage might be and always assuming that the person has passed through it already.

I acknowledge that this is, of course, an extreme reading, exploiting the allowed-for variability of bereavement experiences to the extent where there is no apparent pattern. However, if bereavement experiences *are* like this, then it would be an injustice to fit such experiences to *any* model. The problem is that, according to the majority of bereavement researchers (and even those working within the framework of the biopsychosocial model!), this degree of variability is common. Indeed, the model retains its universality only at the expense of importing *post hoc* explanations to the point at which it becomes modified to a level that compromises any falsifiability (see, for example Kline 1988). This seems hardly consistent with Lofland's (1985: 181) call for 'a willingness to replace sweeping generalizations about grief with its careful and delimited depiction'. The biopsychosocial model of bereavement is neither careful nor delimited; it is vague, of doubtful diagnostic and prognostic value and, in many cases, is an inappropriate way of viewing the experience of bereaved people.

Thus we have a model that is methodologically inconsistent and theoretically incoherent. However, rather than taking the radical step of abandoning a model which is so clearly compromised, practitioners have tended to retain it 'as a set of guidelines'. Indeed, in the absence of any serious competing analysis, the biopsychosocial model would appear to be far too well sedimented in training and practice to be easily dislodged. But is this in the best interests of those to whom it is applied, those people who have been bereaved? I would argue that the answer to this is a very definite 'no'.

First, the promulgation of this model, even only as a system of guidelines, may problematize the experience of the bereaved person. No matter how flexibly the model is used, there is an ever-present danger that the bereaved person takes it literally. Self-help books are now to be found alongside 'academic' texts on bereavement in most major bookshops and this makes it very easy for a bereaved person to begin reading about their experience. What will happen when they read about 'symptoms' of grief which they themselves have not experienced (Lake 1984; Youngson 1989)? How will they feel when they read about the 'stages of grief' (Boston and Trezise 1988; Youngson 1989) and realize that they did not pass through one or more of these stages? Does this mean they have not really 'worked through' their grief (Wambach 1985)? Does this mean they did not really love the person who has died because they have not experienced the full gamut of emotions that 'normal' people experience?

What I am saying, then, is that the biopsychosocial model of bereavement carries with it implications of norms against which bereavement experiences can be compared. Any perceived differences can then lead to concerns over the normality of the individual's experience; at this point, we are in the position where the model has potentially marginalized those whom it is meant to serve.

The normalizing properties (Henriques *et al.* 1984) of this model can also be carried through to the counselling situation. It has been argued that those involved in counselling bereaved individuals must be aware of their assumptions about the nature of grief if they are not to fall into rigid, inflexible ways of relating to those with whom they work Hawkins (1989) rightly argues that all counselling, including bereavement counselling, is based on one or more theoretical and explanatory models of experience. Although practitioners are continually reminded of the need for flexibility and awareness in drawing on models of counselling and bereavement, there is an ever-present danger for the inexperienced worker that, in a 'real' and/or difficult counselling situation, it is safer to fall back onto the familiar ground offered by a theoretical model. The model may provide a means for structuring and guiding the counselling relationship, but it also implies both typical and problematic responses to bereavement (Hawkins 1989). Falling back on the model can limit the counsellor's ability to be open to his or her client's experience and, in consequence, can then limit his or her ability to acknowledge/accept the diversity of that experience (Hawkins 1989).

Why, then, has this biopsychosocial model of bereavement responses been retained for so long if, as I have argued, it is fraught with the difficulties highlighted so far. We can shed some light on this issue if we take a step into the realms of social constructionist theory. Broadly speaking, a social constructionist analysis would suggest that what we take to be 'reality' is the product of a continuing process of construction and reconstruction through social interaction (Berger and Luckmann 1967). As far as bereavement responses are concerned, the 'grief reaction' concept has been created and sustained through the construction and re-construction of shared beliefs by professional reality maintainers (e.g. researchers and practitioners in the area of bereavement), to the point where what began as a concept has become the 'natural' response to bereavement. Wambach (1985) refers to such concepts as 'social constructs'; that is, 'an invention which is created among social members and continues to be useful because it explains that which is not readily understood' (p.201). So we can see *why* the biopsychosocial model has become so widely accepted – it is seen as providing an explanatory model of bereavement experiences. However, the arguments put forward here suggest that in fact the model does not serve this purpose and has outlived any usefulness which it may have been deemed to have when originally developed. If anything, the model merely complicates an extremely complex experience even further.

As we have seen, bereavement responses are *not* readily understood even now. The 'grief reaction' concept does not constitute a theory of 'what happens following bereavement'; it merely describes that which individuals report as having been their experience. As Archer and Rhodes (1987: 212) argue: 'this [grief reaction] provides more of a description than an explanation of underlying processes', and as such does not provide any insight into 'grief' itself.

However, questioning the plausibility of the biopsychosocial model of bereavement responses does not deny the subjective reality of such experiences to those who voice them. What it does do is to challenge the taken-for-grantedness of socially sedimented concepts such as the 'grief reaction'. Without such a challenge this 'disorderly collection' of 'symptoms' (Cochran and Claspell 1987) is sustained and perpetuated, taking on the mantle of objective truth despite its 'impoverished and somehow inaccurate' appearance (Hoagland 1983).

What happens now? If we reject the biopsychosocial model for the reasons given, what do we put in its place? How do we understand bereavement responses without reference to such a model? In order to address these questions, we need to remain a little longer within the realms of social constructionism. This approach provides an alternative understanding of emotional experiences that rejects the need to search for 'essences' and 'universals'. In contrast to the essentialist practitioner, the social constructionist regards the bereaved person's account/report of their experience as a 'gestalt' rather than as a collection of 'symptoms', suggesting that the individual's experience can only be intelligible when accepted as such. This is not to deny that commonalties may emerge between individuals' accounts, if only because individuals share similar (though never identical) socially constructed worlds, but no attempt is made to extrapolate such commonalties to a 'model of grief', or to raise them to the status of universal characteristics or 'symptoms' of grief. In rejecting the aim of discovering 'the essence of grief', the social constructionist practitioner also challenges/rejects the primacy ascribed to that essence by biopsychosocial explanations of bereavement. Thus, this alternative understanding of bereavement responses no longer presupposes an intervening essential griefness upon which individual and social factors exert their influence. Such a 'leap' would be inconsistent with the social constructionist understanding that takes accounts *as* experience, rather than as a means of inferring the nature of some assumed inner state.

A brief visit into the sphere of religious debate at this point provides an analogy that both illustrates this situation and suggests a possible alternative. Almost 20 years ago, the concept of a 'Copernican revolution' was 'borrowed' from the field of astronomy as a way of addressing the controversy surrounding the relationship between Christianity and other world religions. Hick (1976) argued that the invocation of such a revolution would help to resolve the issue of 'conflicting truth-claims' within the major world religions. Hick's response to this problem, as with the original Copernican Revolution, was to shift the focus around which everything revolves. In the case of religion, this would mean focusing on God, ultimate reality, etc., rather than on any particular religious belief system. As Hick (1976: 125) himself comments:

> . . . the Ptolemaic theology [is that] whose fixed point is the principle that outside the church . . . there is no salvation. When we find men of other faiths we add an epicycle of theory to the effect that although they are consciously adherents of different faiths, nevertheless they may unconsciously or implicitly be Christians. In theory, one can carry on such manoeuvres indefinitely.

At first glance, the relevance of Hick's argument may appear somewhat abstruse. However, this conflict situation can be seen to parallel the conflict arising from the competing truth-claims of bereavement researchers. Restating Hick's comments, *but with the addition of the phrases in parentheses*, serves to highlight the corresponding problem in the field of bereavement research and practice:

> . . . the Ptolemaic theology [is that] whose fixed point is the principle that outside the church [*the biopsychosocial model*] . . . there is no salvation [*truth/knowledge*]. When we find men of other faiths [*other patterns of bereavement experience*] we add an epicycle of theory to the effect that although they are consciously adherents of different faiths [*variations from the model*], nevertheless they may unconsciously or implicitly be Christians [*accommodated to the model with a few post hoc modifications*]. In theory, one can carry on such manoeuvres indefinitely.

In grief research, it would entail shifting the focus away from the biopsychosocial model, around which everything revolves and within which everything must be accommodated, to the bereavement experience itself and however it is expressed by the individual. Hence, the following comments from Hick (again with analogous aspects of grief research being placed in parentheses):

> It involves a shift from the dogma that Christianity [*that the biopsychosocial model*] is at the centre to the realisation that it is God who [*the*

individual's experience that] is at the centre, and that all the religions [*expressions of the experience*], including our own, serve and revolve around him [*that experience*].

(Hick 1976: 131)

But how do we do this? How do we move the focus directly onto individual experience and away from the influence of the 'belief system' provided by the biopsychosocial model of bereavement? So far, we have seen how the adoption of a biopsychosocial model of bereavement experiences has led to tensions arising at both the theoretical and practical levels of operation. We have also seen how these tensions can be 'eliminated' by viewing such experiences from the alternative, social constructionist perspective. What then of the bereaved client? How does/would this alternative explanation affect their experience in a bereavement counselling relationship? Is it possible for the counsellor to work *without* the guidelines and structure provided by the biopsychosocial model? How do we move the focus directly onto the 'bereavement account' and away from the 'bereavement account in the context of bereavement models'?

Anderson and Goolishian (1992) seem to be echoing these questions in their suggestion of the need for a 'not-knowing' approach within the context of the therapeutic situation: 'not-knowing requires that our understandings, explanations, and interpretations in therapy not be limited by prior experiences or theoretically formed truths, and knowledges' (p.28).

But how can this pre-conceptual way of working be put into practice within the context of bereavement counselling? That is, how can social constructionist theory be relevant/applied to the real world? One way is simply through raising awareness. Even if the practitioner does not 'take on board' constructionist explanations of bereavement responses, the very process of being made aware of tensions within the biopsychosocial approach will increase awareness of their own practice.

This raising of awareness can be taken even further, to the extent of developing a radically different way of working within the counselling situation. This involves approaching 'each clinical experience from the position of not-knowing' (Anderson and Goolishian 1992). Anderson and Goolishian are suggesting a way of working that is consistent with the theoretical position offered by a social constructionist analysis of bereavement responses. In arguing for the abandonment of any 'search for regularities and common meaning that may validate the therapist's theory but invalidate the uniqueness of the client's stories' (p.30), they are arguing for the abandonment of models of experience (including the biopsychosocial model) which 'close [the therapist] to the full meaning of the client's description of their experience' (ibid.).

In conclusion, a review of the current situation in bereavement research and practice suggests that the continued adoption and imposition of a

biopsychosocial model of bereavement responses serve not only to compli-
cate an already complex experience but, more importantly, has potentially
serious consequences for both client and practitioner. It has been argued
that there is an urgent need to *stop modelling* and to *stop tidying up* bereavement experiences. Only then can the acknowledged diversity and rich-
ness of such experiences be given full expression, and be addressed as a
strength rather than as an 'inconvenience' to be overcome through a never-
ending process of research.

The implications of abandoning the biopsychosocial model have also
been considered briefly, particularly with reference to the logistics of counselling without the guidance (safety?) of a theoretical framework. This issue
is now being addressed by those working in the area of 'the social construction of therapy', which, although in its relative infancy as far as practical application is concerned, offers a potentially fruitful area for further
exploration.

Part 3

Towards integration

Introduction

Part 3 of this book is concerned with narratives that might be constructed to make sense of the tensions and resolve the conflicts that exist between different approaches to generating knowledge, and the stresses between the different forms of explanation for health and illness that result.

Neil Cooper and Chris Stevenson begin Chapter 10 on health research by carefully setting out the underpinning philosophy of different inquiry positions. They look explicitly at what each assumes with regard to how we know (epistemology) and what can be known (ontology). According to Neil and Chris, the bodies of knowledge produced by the different inquiry positions are of a specific kind and each aligns more closely with some professional orientations than others. Sometimes, health professionals who choose to research can simply take a disciplinary position and research according to the well-defined inquiry position. However, a more interesting issue concerns what happens when professionals try to do research that cuts across paradigms. In other words, what are the tensions that arise when health researchers try to do research that encompasses the quantitative research methods of biomedicine *and* the qualitative research strategies that have emerged within sociology and psychology?

Neil and Chris keep the 'real world' in sight by acknowledging that, despite these inquiry paradigms being epistemologically distinct and lying in a tense relationship to each other because each entails different criteria for the legitimacy of knowledge, somehow the inherent tensions have been massaged. It is noted that researchers and practitioners do manage the tensions. For example, in their research they have used the different approaches simultaneously. However, such alliances are often uneasy.

Neil and Chris imply that although the modes of inquiry are irreconcilable at a philosophical level, meaningful dialogue between research positions may be established. They argue that post-modern dissatisfaction with positivism has allowed different criteria for what constitutes 'good' research, and in addressing the question of what constitutes 'good' research a dialogue may be opened up. The adoption of a reflexive position in relation to undertaking research facilitates researchers working within any paradigm to set out why the strategies they employ are appropriate to the subject under investigation. Then all research may be judged by the extent to which the researcher reflects of the process of the production of knowledge.

In this way, researchers may acknowledge and comprehend why a particular research method is used, and how appropriate it is for the research aims, thereby establishing a context for assessing how 'good' research transcends the boundaries of the actual inquiry positions.

Similarly, in Chapter 11, Stewart Forster and Chris Stevenson identify that there are tensions between the biopsychosocial model and holism as a means of explaining health and illness. For Stewart and Chris, the tensions between the biopsychosocial model and holism arise as the biopsychosocial model seeks to reduce the complexity of phenomena, while holism creates the impetus to expand understandings. They suggest that personhood is not captured in the biopsychosocial by the collection of the three disciplines, while holism *is* 'everything to do with' the person. As a result of this difference, within the biopsychosocial model people are reduced down to well-defined elements. Conversely, holism celebrates the diversity of people's experience. Stewart and Chris accept that while the biopsychosocial model is a reductionist approximation to holism, it is a useful tool in health care practice. Conversely, holism is difficult to utilize as a tool, because it is difficult to apprehend, yet a good way to think about people.

The apparently paradoxical but pragmatic use of different positions in health care and research is more understandable in the light of the chapter's conclusions. Stewart and Chris suggest that the biopsychosocial model be 'enhanced' with an holistic framework that consists of practitioners adopting holistic or humane thinking. With this framework in place, practitioners will not be so constrained by professional socialization, but will draw on a wide range of knowledge sources. Using an holistic or humane perspective, practitioners will gain more flexibility in their practice in relation to understanding the health and illness of the persons concerned.

With their discourse, Chapters 10 and 11 set the backdrop for the final chapter. Chris Stevenson and Neil Cooper draw upon the ideas about inquiry positions and holism in establishing how explanations which are hierarchically arranged may nevertheless be 'integrated', at least in an alternative sense. They argue that holism may be defined as simply an extra superior layer added to a biopsychosocial hierarchy of explanations. However, because holism is a concept, rather than an element, it can set a context in which the articulations between the biological, psychological and social can be coordinated and given meaning.

10

Health research

Neil Cooper and Chris Stevenson

Introduction

In research, there are many different ways of approaching health-related issues. Each academic discipline is associated with specific forms of knowledge generated through particular research strategies. This knowledge is then incorporated into professional practice. The research strategies are underpinned by different philosophical positions that are irreconcilable. This chapter looks for ways in which 'common ground' between research positions can be found.

Rather than attempting integration at the philosophical level, it will be argued that one way of reconciling research positions is through the activity of the researchers themselves, and in particular through the criteria which they utilize to determine what is 'good' research. First, however, the chapter sets out three main inquiry positions that can be taken in relation to health. It argues that the methodology of an inquiry position generates knowledge of a specific kind. It is suggested that inquiry positions and disciplinary approaches are related, and that the process of generating knowledge serves to reaffirm the boundaries of disciplines and the research position itself. While specific professional roles cannot easily be placed within the inquiry positions, the chapter will illustrate how professional perspectives may draw explicitly and implicitly upon the different inquiry positions, and that such relations may be important in defining professional views and the research undertaken within professions.

The chapter then assesses whether any criteria for 'good' research exist that would overarch different research positions. Through critiques of positivism, constructivism and social realism, the potential of researcher 'reflexivity' as a criterion for assessing health research is introduced. It is also proposed that such reflexivity, if utilized by practitioners engaged in research, will augment the potential for holistic practice.

Three inquiry positions

A variety of inquiry positions can be taken in relation to health and health care research. Moon *et al.* (1991) suggested that all inquiry positions lie along a continuum that has positivism at one end and constructivism at the other. Positivism, in the context of this chapter, is defined as the position that all knowledge is held within the bounds of science, and that a real world can be objectively observed/measured. Science leads to the development of laws, which can be logically linked together to form theories. Constructivism, in the context of this chapter, is defined as the position that all knowledge arises from the ideas held individually and collectively by social actors. Consequently, objective observation is impossible. Constructivism is a global term that encompasses, but is not synonymous with, social constructionism. Social constructionism is the position that the 'real' world is co-created through conversation. Constructivism includes the position that an individual actor's ideas structure his or her world. For example, Hoffman gives an example of how our ideas organize our experience:

> I have a sea shell collection. I keep it scattered on beaches all over the world.' A sea shell on a beach is a part of an ecosystem. Add the collector who is speaking, and you have the missing element – the idea in the mind of a person about beaches and shells and their relationship to each other and to her.
>
> (Hoffman 1985: 383, quoting the comedian Steve Wright)

Moon *et al.* (1991) pointed out that, according to its position on the continuum, any inquiry stance will entail certain suppositions concerning epistemology (how we know) and ontology (what can be known). If, for example, a positivist health researcher wanted to know about teenage pregnancy, he or she might develop a questionnaire to canvas teenage attitudes and behaviour in relation to unprotected sex. The assumption is that the questionnaire, administered by the distant researcher, would capture the real world of teenagers' sexual activity. Conversely, a constructivist researcher might gather together a group of teenagers in order to have a discussion about their views on unprotected sex, the assumption being that the conjoint discussion between the 'close-up' researcher and teenagers will lead to a co-construction concerning the meanings of unprotected sexual behaviour.

Moon and co-workers (1991) offered a third inquiry position on their continuum, that of post-positivism. Post-positivism is consistent with critical realism (Guba 1990). Critical realism, and post-positivism, accept that there is a world 'out there', but it cannot be represented accurately because of the limits of human perception and cognition. The world can only be known imperfectly. Absolute objectivity is not possible, because the observer necessarily influences the observed. However, modified objectivism is feasible. Stevenson (1995b) has suggested that a post-positivist position is consistent with *social* realism as well as critical realism. Social realism involves modified objectivity, rather than the absolute objectivity which strict positivists claim. Yet the complete merging of the researcher with the researched, which pure constructivist research entails, is neither sought nor attained. A social realist position avoids the pitfalls of taking an extreme position:

> . . . on the one hand, the seductions of objectivity with its myth of dispassionate non-engagement in which the observer is unobserved; and on the other hand, the seductions of becoming a participant in the activity, accepting a prefigured role and only reinforcing the pattern. The former is a mystification, the second a captivation.
>
> (Pearce 1992: 159)

A social realist who is researching teenage pregnancy might undertake semi-structured interviews with teenagers. The accounts will be taken as reflective of an underlying *social* reality, which is accessible by the researcher when he or she analyses the accounts. The analysis will not involve the assumption that the real world of teenage behaviour has been captured, as in positivism. Neither will the researcher seek meanings of sexual behaviour that emerge through the process of the research itself. Rather, the researcher will seek the shared reality of teenage sexual behaviour mediated through the lens which the teenagers themselves apply.

The inquiry positions and bounded knowledge

Shotter (1986) described three different kinds of knowledge that arise from research: (1) *knowledge-that*, theoretical knowledge concerning a phenomenon; (2) *knowledge-how*, knowledge that is applied in practice; and (3) *knowledge-from*, 'insider' knowledge that comes into existence through the process of the research. These qualitatively different kinds of knowledge may be linked to specific inquiry positions (Stevenson 1995a). Put differently, the meaning of the research often emerges from the methodology. Knowledge-that and knowledge-how are linked to positivism and social realism, in which ontology – or what can be known – is of foremost concern. Knowledge-from is linked to constructivism, in which epistemology – or how we know – is the focus.

When a research paradigm has a well-defined position in relation to how we know and what can be known, and the methods which can be used in the pursuit of knowledge, it has a methodology. In the context of this chapter, quantitative methods are associated with positivist research approaches and qualitative methods with research positions nearer to, but not co-terminus with, the constructivist end of Moon and co-workers' (1991) continuum. Social realism is associated with both methods of data collection.

Methodologies tend to be self-sustaining and self-serving. For example, positivists will 'do' research following their particular research 'recipe'. The results of the research will be read by a similarly oriented community, who will judge the research in terms of specific, well-agreed, shared criteria. The self-sustaining nature of methodology is equally apparent within research taking a more constructivist stance, or within social realism. For example, Atkinson *et al.* (1991), taking a broadly constructivist perspective, suggested that research should be evaluated by the community of stakeholders, the consumers of the research. The stakeholders have, by definition, a vested interest in maintaining a specific kind of knowledge and so are likely to keep the boundaries around the research intact. The self-sustaining process of knowledge production means that a certain kind of knowledge is always produced. The criticism is similar to that made by Moon *et al.* (1991), that Kuhnian paradigms are self-sustaining because of the vested interests of a paradigm's defenders.

Methodology may also preserve professional boundaries. The disciplines of biology, psychology and sociology, which underpin our understanding of health, have developed applied fields to varying degrees. The biological approaches, such as physiology, microbiology and immunology, find an applied expression in medicine and may be considered as valuing the positivist position, with methods oriented around quantitative data collection. Medicine's deep linkages with positivistic science maintains the profession's integrity, proficiency and perceived efficacy.

Sociology also has positivist traditions. For example, Durkheim (1897/1970) used empirical techniques in his analysis of social structure to explore suicide. However, sociology has not developed an *explicitly* applied field. While positivist traditions are evident, sociology may be more strongly linked with constructivism and qualitative strategies.

Professions such as social work, in which the ideology of user empowerment is very strong (Biehal and Sainsbury 1991), can draw upon the qualitative strategies emerging in the social sciences. Adopting such a research position enables the social worker to undertake research that reflects the ethos of the profession. The use of qualitative methodologies is also apparent in nursing research.

In contrast to sociology, psychology has developed applications in several specific areas, with clinical and health psychology being major aspects. Within psychology, allegiance to methodologies may be varied:

> . . . psychology appears to lack the coherence of the sciences it takes as its models. It is divided into rival and competing schools – functionalism,

gestalt psychology, psychoanalysis, physiological psychology. One might almost regard each as having a distinct paradigm, each conceiving of its objects and problems differently, utilising different explanatory schemes and conducting different types of research.

(Rose 1985: 221)

The suggestion is that the world view of the researcher is intimately related to the type of research being undertaken. While early researchers in psychology, such as Wundt in the 1870s and James in the 1890s, modelled psychological investigations on natural sciences, they argued that social phenomena were not reducible to more elementary processes (Bornstein 1984). Despite this, in the nineteenth century, psychology shifted from philosophy to experimental research methods, and has since in general attempted to establish itself within a 'scientific' framework. It is this 'scientific' model that has been largely accepted by medicine, especially with respect to the links between psychological variables and specific diseases. In their application, the 'scientific' aspects of psychology have given rise to the need for specific standards and quality of research practice in order to maintain the perceived professionalism of applied psychologists (Elton-Wilson 1992; Lindley and Bromley 1995). The allegiance to objective methods of inquiry maintains 'scientific' respectability and promotes the professionalism of psychologists. However, constructivist approaches are increasingly being employed, especially in psychological investigations which seek to understand social problems and health (Henwood and Nicholson 1995). These alternative methodologies create a particular form of knowledge that challenges the nature of the discipline of psychology itself.

Positivist science, with its emphasis on the experimental method, has also been closely related to masculine investigation, and the medical profession may be considered a patriarchal system. Feminist research has strongly favoured qualitative, constructivist approaches (e.g. Orr 1986). The qualitative research strategies currently employed in nursing and social work may be related to the feminine associations of these professions. This indicates that the expression of human knowing is connected to cultural patterns.

Given the cultural supremacy of the positivist approach to science, it is not surprising that the knowledge created within medicine is associated with power, with the other (female) professions positioned as secondary 'allies' to medicine. The different research approaches therefore have implications for how professions are developed and maintained, and what form of disciplinary knowledge they draw upon.

Perhaps because of the potentially far-reaching consequences for disciplines and professions of adopting a qualitative inquiry position, the legitimacy of qualitative research is frequently questioned by the research establishment. When researchers and professionals who favour a specific inquiry paradigm have the opportunity to evaluate research that is based on different epistemological assumptions, they nevertheless use their own criteria of 'good' research. Understandably, research that is based on a different inquiry position is usually seen as methodologically inadequate. Through the process of denying the validity of research based on different positions, methodological boundaries are firmly maintained. Take, for example, the process of going through a hospital research committee, consisting mainly of medically oriented practitioners and researchers, with a proposal to evaluate an approach to psychotherapy with a constructivist methodology. The research applicant will be in a disadvantaged position unless he or she can engage with the research language of the dominant medical model, either by 'selling out' or finding ways to re-language qualitative methods so that they do not transgress quantitative standards of reliability/validity. A common means of satisfying the requirements is to present a quantitative design with a qualitative design to run in parallel within the project.

Integrating research methods

When strongly defined methodological positions exist, the possibility of integrating research perspectives is daunting. In an extensive review of the possibility of integrating quantitative and qualitative research, Bryman (1988) concluded that the insistence of the researchers entrenched within the two camps that the two approaches are distinct has fuelled the argument that they are not commensurable at an epistemological level. At a practical level, however, there are many examples of quantitative and qualitative approaches being utilized simultaneously.

One means to avoid the integration question is to step outside it and think of some overarching criteria for what constitutes 'good' research. In order to assess the possibility of developing overarching criteria for what constitutes good research, some of the assumptions currently held by researchers taking different inquiry positions need to be explored.

The problems of positivist and constructivist research

A growing dissatisfaction with positivism has been charted in academic literature for several decades and in several scientific and professional fields. For example, the Frankfurt School, a Marxist intellectual movement active from the 1920s until the 1950s, which included Horkheimer, Adorno, Fromm and Marcuse among its members, considered that the quantifiable information produced from a positivist standpoint only scratched the surface of social life and did not develop in-depth sociological analysis.

Laing (1960: 24), writing from an anti-psychiatry perspective, stated:

If it is held that to be unbiased one should be 'objective' in the sense of depersonalising the person who is the 'object' of our study, any temptation to do this under the impression that one is thereby being scientific must be rigorously resisted. Depersonalisation in a theory that is intended to be a theory of persons is as false as schizoid depersonalisation of others and is no less ultimately an intentional act. Although conducted in the name of science, such reification yields false 'knowledge'.

In the field of family therapy, the 1980s saw a review of models of family functioning in which the therapist worked on the family to produce an improvement or cure. The dominant model was linked closely to positivism (Frugerri and Matteini 1988). Maturana and Varela (1980) asserted that the observer has a role in relation to the production of knowledge. Their idea was warmly embraced by many family therapists, who were aware that they were situated within the family system and were not external 'fixers'.

Atkinson *et al.* (1991) denied the value of the researcher justifying his or her approach, whether quantitative or qualitative, by drawing on positivist criteria. Rather, as Walters (1990: 461) asserted, 'there is no predictable blueprint that regulates the pattern of discovery'. Henwood and Pidgeon (1992) have suggested that to be constrained to positivist justification is to ignore the role of imaginative and intuitive qualities of the researcher. Their point is echoed in the opinions of Atkinson *et al.* (1991: 162):

> It is possible, even likely, that the insights of a bright, imaginative researcher who followed no discernible systematic procedures for observation and note-taking could be of a consistently higher quality, as evaluated by a community of stakeholders than the insights of a task oriented researcher who carefully followed the systematic methods of data gathering.

The critique of positivism has not been solely generated by mental health or social science disciplines. Gould (1981), a palaeontologist, made an articulate attack on the assumptions that positivist researchers make about their work. In essence, he questioned the extent to which the researcher can stand aloof to the research process. He summarized the limitations of positivist research thus:

> I do not deny the power, or the great success, of Cartesianism, but hold that its limits have probably been reached in the explanation of complex historical systems . . . equally powerful (but different) techniques of historical *sciences* – with their themes of irreducible interaction, hierarchy, and resolvable contingency – must be embraced to break the hegemony of what, in our parochialism, we call *the* scientific method . . . with its primary themes of experiment, laboratory control, repetition and quantification.
>
> (Gould 1989: 14)

Gould closely allied positivism, science and the experimental method, each of which distances the researcher from the researched. Practitioners in health care often have improvement and change as a focus of concern, but they are, frequently, preoccupied with evaluating their own practice. A methodology based upon positivism limits the range of such evaluation and a constructivist research position may be a more useful approach. For example, action research around a particular problem in a specific context, which stresses the involvement of those concerned and collaboration between practitioner and researcher (Whyte 1984), may be a useful approach in health research. The strategy is difficult to develop within a positivist framework that requires objectivity. It is more consistent with constructivism. Action research also has a democratic function in relation to the research process (Carr and Kemmis 1986). It is an antidote to the power that resides in the production of positivist research.

But in constructivist research there is no strong methodological position. All research-based knowledge is merely a narrative constructed by the researcher and the researched. Stevenson (1994) used an analogy from *Alice in Wonderland* to illustrate the dangers of research whose only methodological position is that there is no discernible, defined methodology:

> First (the Dodo) marked out a race-course in a rough circle ('the exact shape doesn't matter', it said) and then all the party were placed along the course here and there. There was no 'one, two, three and away!' but they began running when they liked, and left off when they liked, so that it was not easy to know when the race was over. However when they had been running half an hour or so . . . the Dodo suddenly called out 'The race is over!', and they all crowded round it, panting and asking 'But who has won?' This question the Dodo could not answer without a great deal of thought . . . at last [it] said, 'Everybody has won, and all must have prizes'.
>   (The Caucus Race, *Alice in Wonderland* by Lewis Carroll)

The problem is that constructivism deconstructs research positions without offering any reconstructed methodological position. The vacuum arises because of the relativism implicit within constructivism. From a relativist position, all accounts of the world are equally good, and so all research positions are equally good also. Yet even Rorty, himself labelled as a relativist philosopher, acknowledged that some explanations are better than others:

> . . . one cannot find anyone who says that two incompatible opinions on an important topic are equally good. The philosophers who get *called* 'relativists' are those who say that the grounds for choosing between options are less algorithmic than had been thought.
>   (Rorty 1982: 166)

Therefore, although constructivists emphasize that different perspectives are equally valid, this position is difficult to maintain. In the face of the difficulty, constructivist researchers adopt existing approaches that fall at the softer end of inquiry (e.g. grounded theory; Glaser and Strauss 1967), but which fulfil at least some of the requirements of 'good' research from a positivist viewpoint.

Mediating positivism and constructivism: social realism

Social realism seems, at first glance, to offer a compromise between the absolute objectivism of some positivists and the relativism of some constructivists. As Golann stated in relation to family therapy research:

> The rejection of a privileged observational method – one that claims to describe interaction in a theoretically neutral and uniquely correct manner – does not mean that, thereafter, anything goes with regard to description . . . observers make multiple or repeated observations of the same event, or may use subjectivity to enrich observation. It follows that we should not dismiss the possibility of a relatively accurate description of a family in interaction.
>
> (Golann 1987: 335)

Within a social realist approach to research, the 'real' world can be known through the shared accounts of the social which participants in events give. It is a position that accepts that the world can be known only imperfectly, but it does not accept that any account is as good as any other. Taking a social realist approach is consistent with 'realism' as defined by Harré (1981). A realist position takes theory as a description of the mechanisms responsible for a pattern of events, or properties of things:

> On the realist view, theories must be the central object of concern in the human sciences. They purport to describe aspects of the world not available to direct experience but generative of it. They are actively involved in the schematising of sensation into perceived fact and in the disambiguating of indeterminate events into socially meaningful actions.
>
> (Harré 1981: 4)

The theory is grounded in, but not limited by, the accounts of participants in events. Stevenson (1995b) argued that grounded theory (Glaser and Strauss 1967) is consistent with social realism.

A social realist position may simply represent a 'watered down' form of positivism. Reason and Rowan (1981) argued that grounded theory seeks to discover real facts within qualitative data. Yet for positivists it does not go far enough, because social realists take the view that reality is mediated through the lenses of actors.

Constructivists might also express a concern that social realism does not go far enough, in that it simply does not give enough consideration to the researcher's role in knowledge production. So while a social realist approach attempts to bridge the divide between positivist and constructivist research, it may represent the worst of both positions.

'Science': reflexivity as an integrative force for researcher/ practitioners

Practitioners, of course, may be researchers as well. The medical profession has a well-established convention of practitioners undertaking research. The tradition is not so well developed as in professions such as nursing and social work which operate more on an academic/practice split.

While practitioners may hold preconceptions about the environment in which they work and may face restrictions due to hierarchical working arrangements, they may also be able to utilize this insider knowledge and practitioner insights, that make research particularly relevant and useful in a specific application. The potential synergy between research and practice means that the integration is beneficial to both (Allen-Meares and Lane 1990).

Winter (1989) considered that as professionals approach their everyday work with a complex number of theories and approaches, the research process – if it is to be useful and offer new insights – must offer something different to practitioners' everyday activities and knowledge. Winter suggested that rather than just applying research processes, practitioners should use them in a reflexive fashion, in a dialectical way. Linking research and practice may facilitate reflexivity about 'caring'. By undertaking research that is utilized in a reflexive way, practitioners are forced into considering both the philosophical aspects of research and the underpinnings of practice. The process may lead to a consideration of alternative ways of looking at specific problems and will maintain a more open and aware mind. Through the process of reflection, more humane or holistic practitioners who are able to value different forms of knowledge will emerge.

Empowering professionals with research tools may facilitate increased reflexivity in their practice, and enable them to appreciate the positions and philosophy which informs their day-to-day work. This suggests that researcher/practitioners may utilize any research position. Bryman (1988) argued that the crucial activity is to choose an inquiry position appropriate to the phenomenon to be researched. The need for careful consideration when choosing a research paradigm is neatly illustrated by a quotation from Keeney (1983: 56–7):

Epistemologist: Let us take an example from our history books. Do you remember reading about a time when people believed that the world was flat? A ship that went too far out into the ocean was believed to drop off the planet. Of course when these ships later returned, people began to believe that our world is circular rather than flat. Photographs of the earth taken from a satellite in outer space now confirm the circular earth hypothesis. Anyone belonging to the Flat Earth Society is seen as being a bit weird.

Therapist: That's a nice metaphor for family therapy. Most therapists today claim to subscribe to a 'circular epistemology' and castigate 'lineal thinkers'. A quick way to draw an indication of right and wrong in my field is to invoke the difference between circular and lineal. I cannot imagine anyone claiming to be lineal any more than I could be serious about someone claiming the world is flat.

Epistemologist: G. Spencer Brown reminds us, however, that the flat earth hypothesis is quite sensible at times. For example, if we wish to build a tennis court, draw a blueprint for a house or navigate across the English Channel, we must use the premise that the earth is flat. I dare you to landscape a soccer pitch with a circular earth hypothesis. On the other hand, if we wish to sail around the world we need to switch to a circular hypothesis.

Although researchers are freed in their choice of research approach, maximum utility occurs when a method is employed in a reflexive fashion; that is, when the position of the researcher is taken into account when considering the research design and findings. This raises the issue that it is how the research is considered rather than the approach itself which is important.

The thesis, developed above, is that research of all kinds involves the researcher's contribution to the phenomenon studied. The need for researcher reflexivity can be used as the underpinning rationale for delimiting at least one important criterion of 'good' research. For example, one way in which research of all kinds might be evaluated is by the extent to which the researcher *reflects* on the choice of his or her inquiry position. The reflection would include a consideration of the epistemological and ontological prejudices that influence choice.

Researcher reflexivity would also involve the researcher considering whether his or her own involvement has enhanced or detracted from the 'findings'. Krippendorf (1991: 133) argued that all researchers are 'discursively constructing the very contexts that render their data meaningful'. Webb (1992) advocated the inclusion of a reflexive stance in research. She also recommended the presentation of the reflexive material to the reader, alongside unedited chunks of data, sufficient for the reader to evaluate the researcher's conclusions. Lincoln and Guba (1985) suggested that the researcher keep a reflexive journal alongside the research process, which should be open to external audit. The suggestion applies to any researcher, student, academic or practitioner, irrespective of their inquiry position.

Conclusion

Inquiry positions can be sited along a continuum with positivism at one extreme and constructivism at the other. Social realism sits midway. Different inquiry positions are associated with different kinds of knowledge. They are not neutral in that they are self-sustaining and self-serving. They often help to preserve disciplinary boundaries, but exceptions occur; for example, in psychology, where an expansion of methodologies challenges the nature of the discipline itself. The recognition of qualitative methods by those disciplines with a quantitative orientation would potentially have similar effects. Yet at a practical level, different methodologies have been applied within research projects. However, the extent to which integration can be claimed is doubtful. The integration may not even be desirable, given that existing inquiry positions have been extensively criticized. A compromise methodology may simply revolve around the worst of two alternatives. A creative definition of science that celebrates the reflexivity of the practitioner/researcher is advocated, alongside an open-minded approach for selecting a suitable methodology. The degree of reflection applied by the researcher becomes the overarching criterion for 'good' research.

11

Holistic thinking: personhood and the biopsychosocial model

Stewart Forster and Chris Stevenson

Introduction

This chapter explores the relationship of the biopsychosocial model to holism. It argues that the biopsychosocial, model is reductionist as it is concerned with rigidly defined parts of the person rather than wholes. Each part offers a different level of explanation of human functioning. Reason (1994: 12) described the process and outcome of compartmentalizing our world as follows:

> . . . the tendency [is] to think in terms of parts rather than wholes, things rather than processes: naming the parts of the world creates an *illusion* (our emphasis) of real separate objects; concepts drive a wedge, as it were, between experience and understanding. These mental constructions, or paradigms, are immensely robust and self-fulfilling when isolated from experience.

The biopsychosocial model assumes that people are a reflection of their biological, psychological and social aspects. These aspects are considered to be interrelated, but are treated in practice as distinct 'levels' of explanation, each with a comprehensive and discrete body of knowledge that practitioners can 'dip into'. We contend that wholes, or some wholes, are more than the sum of their parts. For us, holism refers to *everything to do with* some thing that goes towards its final make-up. These 'things to do with' may not necessarily appear as 'real' or tangible phenomena; for example, they may be ideas or beliefs about objects. The meanings may be constructed by the person him or herself or by the observer. The definition places emphasis on the Gestalt nature of objects. The whole is different from the sum of its parts. The whole arises through the relationships of the parts. For example, people exist through the way in which they present themselves, and through the way in which they are perceived by others. For us, an holistic definition of a person is more than the sum of the parts of the biopsychosocial model. Holism refers to *personhood* as the totality of a person's being embedded in his or her social world.

In this chapter, we consider how the biopsychosocial model is a useful, though reductionist, practice tool operating as a part of hierarchical health care. By hierarchical health care, we mean systems where health care professionals take, or are given, precedence over those who seek help. A review of the biopsychosocial model is undertaken. The model's potential when expanded by systems theory is considered. We conclude that neither of these two positions is holistic because neither is good at considering the whole person. Conversely, we propose that an holistic perspective does provide a useful way to think about people. Yet its complex nature entails difficulties in subsequent application. In the final section, we suggest that holism can provide a conceptual framework that will inform but not dictate practice. We conclude that thinking holistically can liberate practitioners to take different positions in relation to caring activities and join with their patients/ clients in defining problems and solutions.

The biopsychosocial model and a systemic perspective: hierarchical and holarchic health care

Health professionals look for problems (and solutions) that can be explained in terms of the levels of the biopsychosocial model. Assessment and intervention are directed at each level individually. Sometimes a single level is emphasized. This point is made by Chris Stevenson and Phil Barker in Chapter 4, where they describe how professionals divide up their work according to their particular theoretical orientation. For instance, pain is often considered from a physiological perspective, and its management remains largely pharmaceutical in nature. Conversely, anxiety is considered to be a psychological problem and treatment is approached through 'talking therapies'. Sometimes two or more levels are addressed simultaneously; for example, treating depression with anti-depressant medication *and* cognitive therapy. The co-influence of levels is not accounted for. For example, there is no consideration of the biological mechanism that might change in response to the 'talking therapy'; and there is little consideration of how the medication might influence the psyche, beyond a global description of 'mood elevation'.

Practitioners manipulate the biological, psychological and sociological elements of the model in order to arrive at a meaningful model for health care. However, the elements of the biopsychosocial model are manipulated without a full understanding of what each different element represents in terms of the individual as a whole. For example, what is the person's experience of being depressed and treated with medication and cognitive therapy? Consequently, the biopsychosocial model falls short of being holistic. In turn, the treatment plan that arises out of manipulation in this manner cannot be holistic, although it may be perceived by the professional to be so.

The biopsychosocial model involves the professional acting upon the patient or client without much reflexivity about the professional's own position. Reflexivity is perceived as unnecessary given the current focus on the biopsychosocial model. Taking nursing as an example, assessments are completed with the intention of finding problems and devising effective strategies to solve them. Similarly, nursing, practice in the mid-1990s has undergone the introduction of care mapping in which pre-written 'ideal' routes for illness progression, and consequent care needs, are conceived. This style of managing ill health represents a trend whereby professionals are required to think little about exploring and modifying care needs. Essentially, the patient's or client's view on the relevance of professional knowledge is not sought. In Foucault's (1975) terms, there is a knowledge hierarchy sustained by the exclusivity of professional discourse. Patients/clients perceive that practitioners are knowledgeable experts. The perception helps to maintain practitioners in a powerful position as far as providing treatment is concerned. So, for example, the current ethos within nursing and medicine is that nurses and doctors simply 'know best'. Nurses and doctors have implicit power (Stevenson 1995b).

Such hierarchical systems emphasize that health is, or can be, achieved via the replacement of 'bad' health behaviours with 'good' ones, on the advice of the 'knowing' health care professional. Seedhouse (1991) has discussed the role of indoctrination in health education, and how it has proscribed patient/client choice within health care settings:

> Indoctrination undermines the *central conditions* that people should have the fullest possible information about factors which affect their lives, and that they should have sufficient ability and range of information to make their own reasoned choices.
>
> (Seedhouse 1991: 84)

Professionals intervene in people's lives in order to make them better according to the professional definition. Their activity is not neutral. As Bloor and McIntosh (1990) suggested, when professionals inquire into the parts of a person's life which that person does not want or believe it useful to explore, they are exercising a political function of surveillance. It is not acceptable to categorize patient/client problems on a global basis, drawing on the biopsychosocial or any other model without the person's agreement. Categorization in this form is not consistent with individualized care or individualized health belief models, much less holism.

While the biopsychosocial model explains phenomena at discrete levels, the different aspects *are* related, as Engel (1977) argued. For instance, treating particular problems with specific conventional treatments may well affect the individual at more than one level. However, the effect at a different level is not part of an intentional act on the part of health care professionals – it may not even be recognized. Consider the effects of a referral to an occupational therapist made on behalf of someone who knows that they are not coping adequately with daily activities at home. The mere knowledge that a referral has been made and his or her 'case' discussed may reduce stress and increase psychological well-being for that person. However, within the area of practice, the problem remains under the banner of 'the social', and the associated benefits are scarcely considered at all. The action of the professional cannot be considered as actively treating more than one level of the problem.

Engel (1977) considered that superimposing systems theory on to the biopsychosocial model would allow more comprehensive understandings of phenomena. Systems theory involves the position that change in one level necessarily effects change in other associated levels. For instance, certain lifestyles are said to be associated with stress. The subsequent changes within biology (e.g. high levels of glucocorticoids) predispose the individual to illnesses, such as coronary heart disease and cerebral vascular accident. Similarly, biological illness itself can result in a variety of reactions, not only from society at large, but within the psychological response of the individual. For example, the labelling of a person as psychiatrically ill, with the assumption of some biological disturbance, has an effect on their self-esteem, their perceived level of control, and so on, within a society where mental illness is stigmatized. According to Engel (1977: 134), the adoption of a systems approach 'should do much to mitigate the holist–reductionist dichotomy'. An examination of a different health care arrangement helps to demonstrate Engel's position.

'Holarchy' (Koestler 1964; Scaife 1993) represents a position distinct from hierarchical arrangements within which the biopsychosocial model operates. It is consistent with a systems theory approach as advocated by Engel (1977). In an holarchy there is respect for both the individual system (the person) and the wider system (society). Individual systems can adopt the position of looking inwards or outwards in relation to other systems or parts. The notion is closely tied in with the concept of Holons (Koestler 1964). Everything is both an element of something else (looking out) and a whole thing in its own right (looking in). For instance, tissues, organs, anatomical groups and people all constitute systems in their own right, when 'looking in'. Yet they are also part of greater systems, societies, nations and worlds. The systemic approach of holarchy involves the concept of looking in either direction *ad infinitum*, and it is because of this that the biopsychosocial model is a poor approximation to holarchy. The biopsychosocial model is an inflexible model that does not currently match with the notion of an holarchy that stretches infinitely in both 'directions', and implies the possibility of many different positions and perspectives. Thus, the biopsychosocial model does not fit with holarchy because each level of explanation within the model is treated as a discrete entity (although, as mentioned earlier, treatment in this way is inadequate).

When viewed from an holarchic perspective, the constituent parts of the biopsychosocial model are 'mini' systems in their own right, and contain smaller systems within them (e.g. a chemistry input to biology). These mini systems may then combine to form wider systems (i.e. a psychological input into sociology). For example, we can choose to see a person with a fractured leg as defined by their biological system, in terms of trauma to a particular part of the skeletal frame and the loss of mobility this implies. We can also see the fracture as defining, *and being defined within*, a social relationship, say with a carer, in that the fracture provides an opportunity for the carer to demonstrate their commitment to the person with the fracture. Looking further outward, the caring relationship may itself be part of a specific cultural practice within which the sick are attended to.

We do not find within the application of the biopsychosocial model much exploration of systems. It is not 'normal' for professional interventions to be based upon looking inwards and outwards. There may be a very good reason for this omission. There are, and must be, practical limitations within the clinical area. For example, nursing staff are unlikely to need to explore the national or international consequences of a fracture in planning care for the majority of individuals. Such an expansionist view would include issues largely meaningless in terms of day-to-day management. Moreover, we think that this demonstrates a fundamental problem with a systems theory analysis. Personhood, which we treat as synonymous with holism, is lost as it is subsumed within ever higher levels of systemic organization.

The failure on the part of health care professionals to acknowledge the interrelationship of the distinct levels of the biopsychosocial model is contextualized by relevant research and theory. Some life and physical scientists believe that eventually 'higher'-level phenomena (e.g. a person's psychological experience), will be reducible to biology, chemistry or physics. As the time for this is some way off, it is perfectly legitimate meanwhile to make each level an academic and practice focus. But if, for example, psychology is reduced to chemical processes, to neural events, then it simply becomes chemistry and not psychology. Bateson (1972: 407) pointed out that both co-influence and the distinctness of levels should be recognized:

Now let me begin to talk about the individual organism . . . and its controls are represented in the *total* mind . . . But the system is segmented in various ways, so that the effects of something in your food life, shall we say, do not totally alter your sex life, and things in your sex life do not totally change your kinesic life, and so on.

However, if bodies of knowledge are *rigidly* separated, if an interface cannot be found that respects the difference of the positions while allowing their novel interactive potential, then there is no way in which the biopsychosocial model can be regarded as integrated. We can use an analogy between the biopsychosocial model and parallel lines. The lines never meet. However, if we imagine parallel lines drawn on a piece of paper, by using perspective they can and do meet 'in the distance'. But the use of perspective is an illusory device, similar to the illusion that the biopsychosocial model is holistic. *Real* links between the parallel lines, or levels of explanation, are required.

So far, we have considered the biopsychosocial model as a reductionist approach to health care practice. When the concept of holism is explored further, the division we have drawn between holism and the biopsychosocial model becomes more distinct.

Comprehending holism

Holism is notoriously difficult to apprehend and describe. Holism is all 'organic and fuzzy and warm and cuddly and mysterious' (Dennett 1984: 1453). The following section uses an analogy in order to begin an exploration of holism and relate it to the complex idea of personhood.

Douglas R. Hofstadter (in Hofstadter and Dennett 1981) has implicitly likened holism to a fugue. In the following extract, the Crab, Anteater and Achilles are debating the nature of the fugue, whose quality is difficult to describe or define. Their conversation helps us to think about holism:

Crab: Most definitely. It is quite a tantalising phenomenon, since you feel that the essence of the fugue is flitting about you, and you can't quite grasp all of it, because you can't quite make yourself function both ways at once.

Anteater: Fugues have that interesting property, that each of their voices is a piece of music in itself; and thus a fugue might be thought of as a collection of several distinct pieces of music, all based on one single theme and all played simultaneously. And it is up to the listener (or his subconscious) to decide whether it should be perceived as a unit or a collection of independent parts, all of which harmonise.

Achilles: You say that the parts are 'independent', yet that can't be literally true. There has to be some co-ordination between them, otherwise when they were put together one would just have an unsystematic clashing of tones – and that is as far from the truth as can be.

Anteater: A better way to state it might be this: if you listened to each voice on its own, you would find that it seemed to make sense all by itself. It could stand alone, and is the sense in which I meant that it is independent. But you are quite right in pointing out that each of these individually meaningful lines fuses with the others in a highly non random way, to make a graceful totality . . . this dichotomy between hearing a fugue as a whole and hearing it's component voices is a particular example of a very general dichotomy, which applies to many kinds of structures built up from lower levels.

(Hofstadter and Dennett 1981: 158)

The crab's point is significant to our discussion of holism, in that it is suggestive of the ability to perceive wholes in terms of their separate parts or voices, should we wish. Yet we cannot quite manage to simultaneously appreciate or understand the holistic nature of the overall piece as one unit. The point is restated when the Crab makes a comparison between the fugue and its prelude:

Crab: Yes. Although it may be hard to put it into words, there is always some subtle relation between the two [fugue and prelude; parts and wholes]. Even if the prelude and fugue do not have a common melodic subject, there is nevertheless always some intangible abstract quality which underlies both of them, binding them together very strongly.

(Hofstadter and Dennett 1981: 154)

If we take the example of the fugue and apply it to the biopsychosocial model, the differing and distinct levels present within the biopsychosocial model are represented by the independent voices of the music. The fugue is analogous to an holistic view of persons. The biopsychosocial model fails to account for 'personhood'. Personhood is an emergent property. It emerges out of the relationships between the biology, psychology and sociology of the person and the context provided by the meanings attached to the person by others, as the fugue emerges from the distinct voices. Personhood is an aspect of people not directly reducible to the biological, psychological or social levels. 'Personhood' transcends the sum of the biopsychosocial model.

However, we can understand people as individuals best by dividing them up, by recognizing their different 'voices' or levels of functioning. This is why the biopsychosocial model is a helpful tool, as discussed in the next section.

The biopsychosocial model as a practical tool

The biopsychosocial model does not apprehend 'everything to do with' but sets out those things it can apprehend. The biopsychosocial model categorizes health into the biological, psychological or social realms, which are those aspects of holism it can capture. Consequently, it can be used as a pragmatic method for assessment and intervention without the necessary concentration on the 'everything to do with' that holism entails.

Conversely, for holism to be a useful *tool*, all elements of an entity would have to be apprehensible by observers – and, in health care, manageable. Above, we criticized the biopsychosocial model for its reductionism. For holism to be a *tool*, the 'whole' would in some way have to be added to the parts. We call adding the whole to the parts 'introductionism'. Introductionism is as problematic as reductionism but for the following, different reasons. It is possible to take a position less than holistic, and indeed the biopsychosocial model does so, but it is not possible to take a position that in some way encapsulates holism, within the current biopsychosocial model, in the hope that the biopsychosocial model as a tool will become more comprehensive and/or better. Discussing the mind, Bateson (1972: 408) made a similar point:

> . . . the *whole* mind could not be represented in a *part* of the mind. The television screen does not give you total coverage or report of the events which occur in the whole television process; and this not merely because the viewers would not be interested in such a report, but because to report on any extra part of the total process would require a still further addition of more circuitry, and so on.

People tend to be economical in their cognitive strategies for knowing the world. The above arguments reflect how people simplify complex issues in order to understand and use them. The biopsychosocial model represents an endeavour to represent holism in some way, but because we are unable to represent holism effectively, the biopsychosocial model offers the best available approximation to holism. The biopsychosocial model helps us to narrow or reduce information to make it comprehensible. The biopsychosocial approach can, therefore, be justified as a tool on the basis that it is consistent with, although not synonymous with, an holistic position. However, when complex phenomena are understood in simple terms, errors in judgement and difficulties in getting to grips with phenomena occur. For example, in discussing the concept of 'nothingness', Alice, the March Hare and the Mad Hatter illustrate the potential for 'reality disagreement' (Birch 1994, personal communication) in definitions:

> 'Take some more tea', said the March Hare to Alice very earnestly.
> 'I've had nothing yet', said Alice in an offended tone, 'so I can't take more'.
> 'You mean you can't take less', said the Hatter . . .
>
> (Lewis Carroll, *Alice in Wonderland*)

As argued in the next section, using simplistic concepts to understand people is particularly problematic.

An holistic, heterarchical context for health care

This section presents the argument that holistic thinking provides a context in which the biopsychosocial model can be applied differently. We emphasize the use of holism as a 'new' way of thinking. Thus, holism may be incorporated into the *philosophical* position of practitioners rather than being set as a goal, or assumed to be achievable *within* the biopsychosocial model. For example, thinking holistically would encourage the professional generally to be more flexible and to apprehend the meanings for the client about their situation. Thus, while we have set out the problems of an holistic perspective within health care spheres, we turn now to its positive potential. First, however, we want to argue against *simplistic* versions of holism.

Alternative practitioners claim an holistic approach. Charlton (1993) considered that holism is often associated with alternative practitioners who attempt to utilize personal and social information about their client in an attempt to explain ill health, but rely upon simplistic explanations to do so:

> Thus, every personal and physical detail can be incorporated into an holistic alternative medical system and, in that sense, can be explained. By explaining the complex in terms of the simple, holistic medicine is guilty of being reductionist in the extreme: it explains life in terms of medicine.
>
> (Charlton 1993: 475)

For instance, reflexology, as an alternative therapy, claims to treat the whole individual, but from the position of suggesting that the whole individual is represented by the foot of that individual. We like to label this process 'theoretical shrinking'. Charlton (1993: 475) suggested that 'the goal of holism may be misguided, and instead . . . the humane doctor should be our ultimate aspiration'.

The humane doctor, according to Charlton (1993), will be an individual educated in the arts and liberal studies and have a good general knowledge of how people behave and interact with others. The emphasis needs to be on wisdom as well as skills acquisition, which has dominated medical education and training to date. Distinctions are made here between simplistic holism and humane practice, which are similar to those drawn earlier between the biopsychosocial model and holism as personhood. From this, we conclude that our definition of holism maps well on to Charlton's (1993) description of humane practice, and we use holistic and human practice interchangeably in the remainder of this chapter.

We are, for the greater part, in agreement with Charlton that a common goal should *not* take the form of developing a model that itself strives to be holistic, but settle for a model that 'works' and appreciates the holistic nature of people: a model that is humane. We go on to suggest that underpinning the biopsychosocial model with a humane perspective can lead to a different kind of caring in which patients/clients are empowered in the definition and treatment of their own problems.

In Chapter 7, Nigel Watson urged professionals to listen to lay voices, in order to deconstruct the dominant models of explanation used by professionals. Glynis Hale, in discussing death and dying, suggested that knowledge is socially constructed rather than pre-existing. Knowledge about the patient/client is brought into existence through conversation of patient/client and professional. An holistically, or humanely, oriented professional would, in effect, practise within a framework of negotiation with the patient/client, rather than practise prescriptively within the context of hierarchically based planning. Of prime importance to the holistically oriented practitioner would be the need to encourage the patient/client to express and discuss his or her conceptions with regard to biological, psychological and social health and illness.

The biopsychosocial model, when set in a framework of holism, matches well with Scaife's (1993) idea of heterarchy. Heterarchy is a term used to describe a relationship pattern in which the different participants in an encounter shift their positions over time. The position taken depends on the particular activity engaged in, or topics under discussion. No single person permanently occupies the uppermost position. Each position is unique and respected for its uniqueness. Thus, the health care practitioner working in an heterarchical way will move between the different levels of the biopsychosocial model according to the context.

A health example which contrasts the application of the biopsychosocial model as currently practised and an heterarchical approach to care is helpful in clarifying the differences. Let us take the person identified as having a difficult reaction to bereavement. The biopsychosocial model is often narrowed to a psychological perspective in these circumstances. The professional assumes that the bereaved person must 'work through' specific grief stages, with the help of the professional, in order to adapt to his or her loss. Any biological phenomena (e.g. sleeplessness) are simply assumed to be diagnostic indicators of being stuck in coming to terms with the death. Taking an holistic or humane stance might alter the professional account. The holistic practitioner is interested in the biological, psychological and social aspects of the bereavement process. However, there is no need to treat any one as having precedence over any other. Informed by knowledge of death and dying in our society, gained through social studies, literature, art, and so on, the practitioner's wisdom opens up possibilities for discussing the meanings of different physical, psychological and social aspects of the bereavement process. The discussion means that, instead of being constrained by a ready-made theoretical framework, the practitioner and patient/client can together explore creatively the meanings of bereavement at every level.

Stated differently, when set in an holistic context, it is possible to manipulate the elements of the biopsychosocial model in a way that prevents any one element becoming the dominant focus within the health care setting.

Implicit within the normal movement of conversations between professional and patient/client is the notion that all statements remain relevant as they 'come and go' within the conversation – no attempt is made to regain the focus of one particular level. With an emphasis on the philosophy behind holistic thinking, each facet of the biopsychosocial model becomes *interesting* to the practitioner and patient/client as they construct together the meanings attached to each level of the model. In a sense, the model then becomes integrated. This is not to say that singular treatments are precluded, but an holistic perspective enters into the health care process. It allows those treatments based on a single level of the biopsychosocial model to be surrounded in 'new' thinking.

Conclusion

Wholes, or some wholes, are greater than the sum of their parts. Health professionals assume, in applying the biopsychosocial model, that the three levels of biological, psychological and social represent the whole individual, and act in accordance with this assumption. In particular, professionals assess and treat unilaterally without recourse to the views of their patients/clients about their personal experience. Professional discourse serves to maintain the implicit professional power hierarchy.

The biopsychosocial model is reductionist and overlooks the notion that its levels are related. Systems theory is more attuned to the complex relationship of levels. It is an holarchic position which respects both the individual system and those to which it may contribute. However, neither the biopsychosocial model nor a systems approach accounts adequately for personhood.

The idea that people simplify things in order to understand them better is reflected in claims that the biopsychosocial model is synonymous with holism. Such claims are naive. Exploring the nature of holism crystallizes its differences with the biopsychosocial model. It is suggested that the biopsychosocial model cannot apprehend the holistic nature of a person. It is possible to take a position less than holistic, but it is not possible to take a position that is greater than holism. The addition of extra 'parts' or levels to the biopsychosocial model is introductionist and does not imply movement towards a more holistic position. However, the biopsychosocial model is a pragmatic tool for health professionals.

Holism is not precluded from clinical practice. While it may never become a useful tool, it is a good way to understand people. A 'new' way of thinking within practice is suggested. Holistic or humane thinking can construct a framework to inform practice within the current biopsychosocial model.

The emphasis on holistic thinking as a frame of reference for the biopsychosocial model offers an opportunity within which practitioners might provide more flexible care on a collaborative basis.

12

A reconciling framework

Chris Stevenson and Neil Cooper

Introduction

It is both deeply naive and arrogant to think that the tensions between different levels of explanation of health phenomena can be convincingly reconciled within the pages of one chapter. The preceding chapters have served to demonstrate the range of perspectives on health and the uncertainty about how they relate to one another. Reconciling different levels of explanation is problematic and needs to be respected as such. Yet, there are vague, tantalizing indications of how integration might occur. We hope that the following exploration helps to stimulate academic debate by widening the potential for discourse.

Throughout the chapter, we treat the elements of the biopsychosocial model as distinct forms of explanation for health phenomena. We set out the evidence concerning how different forms of explanation arise, and go on to discuss how their separateness is maintained. We argue for the problematic nature of integrating forms of explanation that are distinct.

We suggest that the different forms of explanation are hierarchically arranged, in that some explanations are seen as more valid or robust than others. In hierarchies of explanation, there is potential for conflict between the levels to occur. For example, as argued throughout the book, medical knowledge based upon biology holds a dominant position in health care. When alternative explanations are put forward, they are denigrated to an inferior position. Within this hierarchical organization of explanations disorder may be created, as the different levels explain the same phenomena using complementary but at the same time contradictory concepts. A simple example to illustrate this idea is the developing infant, who is seen as a product of biological characteristics (nature) *and* the social influences that act on this biology (nurture). While the effect of the social environment may be considered to set a context for biological development (and therefore be complementary to biology), the social world can simultaneously be seen as an explanation in its own right, and this is where confusion arises. We set out different approaches for dealing with confusions. In particular, we look at different theories of how people construct their world in order to make sensible the tangles between levels of explanation. Such attempts at accounting for the confusions may be a productive area in understanding how integration of different explanations could occur.

We conclude with an exploration of one way in which an holistic framework can provide a context within which biological, psychological and social levels can be 'integrated' (in a new sense), as professionals develop 'rules' to help them to make sense of the relationship between those levels and of their own activity.

Forms of explanation

In discussing 'beingness', Laing (1960) argued that wo/man can be seen as a person or a thing. Even the same thing can give rise to two entirely different descriptions, the descriptions give way to entirely different theories, and the theories underpin two different sets of actions. 'The initial way we see a thing determines all our subsequent dealings with it' (Laing 1960: 20). For example, if the depressed person is seen as a thing, psychotropic medication is prescribed; if the depressed individual is seen as a person, then psychotherapy is offered. There is *no* dualism entailed in Laing's position. The different views are not reflective of some underlying split (e.g. a mind–body division). There are not two different essences, the person and the organism at which different treatments are aimed. Rather, they are two different experiential Gestalts. Such different experiential Gestalts may be the basis of different professional world views, each encompassing a form of explanation.

However, many academics do subscribe to dualism, implicitly or explicitly, in their treatment of multiple forms of explanation. Press (1980) used the term 'sympatricity' for a situation in which mutually contradictory theories compete. 'The image is of sympatric theories that operate in parallel, at one and the same time competing and co-existing' (Stainton Rogers 1991: 7). Duality is implied by Press's (1980) exposition. Different theories are concerned with *either* the body *or* the mind. As Chris Stevenson and Phil Barker argue in Chapter 4, a dualist framework helps to account for the ease with which practitioners of different disciplines maintain their own singular world view. Dualism can, therefore, be seen as a force against integration of the biological and psychological and, if we accept another split, the social.

Dualist and non-dualist positions re-converge when integration of explanations is considered. Laing's experiential Gestalts, in common with Press's (1980) co-existing theories, cannot be fully integrated because one explanation cannot become another without losing its own character. Laing (1960) gave the example of listening to another person talking. The listener has the choice of either studying the verbal behaviour as a neural process, or of trying to understand what is being said. Knowing about one aspect does not help in the understanding of the other. In the same way, many separate explanations of health phenomena co-exist. We suspect that there will always be different kinds of explanation defended by theoreticians, who engage in 'good guy/bad guy' discourse about their peers, as each camp considers the other's position as obtuse or callous (Birch 1995). When explanations are given different amounts of credence or status, they may be described as hierarchically arranged.

Hierarchies and integration

The maintenance of different forms of explanation within the biopsychosocial model gives the potential for a hierarchical system of explanation because the forms of explanation are treated as different levels, with the implicit idea that one level can be higher or lower – better or worse – than another. In other words, in making an analysis that distinguishes between the legitimacy of different kinds of knowledge, a hierarchy is necessarily set up.

In general, hierarchical relationships in systems arise when one unit forms the context for interpreting the other. This is the articulation that attempts at integration in the biopsychosocial model have favoured thus far. For example, the intentional level of explanation (i.e. concerning the meanings that people attach to the events that befall them) are often contracted (reduced) to sub-intentional, psychological or biological explanations, or expanded to supra-intentional, social structural explanations.

The hierarchical arrangement of explanations has been implicitly described at several points in the book. For example, the dominance of medical understandings of health has been referred to in terms of its perceived greater status, partly derived from its deep linkages with positivist science, which help to maintain the profession's integrity. More indirectly, biological knowledge is reified through practice; for example, in 'general' nursing, where physical care takes priority over psychological or social needs. The hierarchical division between lay and professional beliefs is also a recurring theme of the book.

In the next section, we argue that hierarchies are a force against integration, because the distinctness of the elements means confusions occur as competing meanings arise when two or more levels are considered simultaneously.

The problematic nature of integration: paradoxes in hierarchical systems of explanation

Once the social scientist accepts the existence of hierarchically organized systems of meaning, he or she must then contend with the structural complexities of hierarchical systems – one of which is the tendency for the systems to exhibit 'tangles' or 'loops' among levels (Cronen *et al.* 1982: 91). The tangles, or loops, are sometimes called reflexive loops, or reflexive paradoxes. The classic example of a reflexive loop is the statement by the Cretan Epimenedes that all Cretans are liars. The problem with such statements is that there are two levels in the system, or communication, and it is unclear which is the higher level. For example, do we accept that Epimenedes is telling the truth when he says all Cretans are liars? If we do, then what position does that leave Epimenedes himself in? Conversely, if we accept that all Cretans are liars, as Epimenedes suggests, then his statement about Cretans lying, on which we have based our assessment, is necessarily false. In other words, competing levels of meaning are set up. Moving upwards and downwards through the levels always has the same outcome. We end up back where we started. Taking an example from practice, the empowerment of clients by professionals may be seen as a mechanism through which 'the client' can achieve greater control over interactions with professionals. As discussed in Chapter 6 in relation to child protection, giving power to others is implicitly a power play, and it can be argued that the client who is the passive recipient of power, therefore, is not actually empowered.

We can also find an example of a 'tangle' or reflexive loop in social science, within which there has been animated discussion concerning the tension between 'the social' and 'the individual'. By focusing in on one discipline's struggle to make itself more academically respectable, we can demonstrate the problems that arise from attempts at integration. In order to become more homogeneous, psychology has attempted a tight definition of its methodology – that is, its aims and organization and methods of inquiry as a discipline. Yet, the attempt has caused more problems for the discipline than it has solved. For example, psychology has been forced to grapple with contradictions between generalist, nomothetic theories about human nature, based on natural science, and more humanistic concerns. The tension has become known as 'Joynson's Dilemma' (Harré 1971), the dilemma being that psychology as a discipline stood in need of the powerful theory, which Joynson (1971) felt had been lacking since the demise of 'positivistic behaviourism'. However, his concern was that such a theory must essentially be physiological in nature and that this would destroy psychology as the discipline that it had become.

Similarly, there is a tension between respecting the individuality of a person's experience and the recognition that shared culture and social experience are important (Stainton Rogers 1991). Is the individual influenced by, or the product of, the social context? Does the individual act on the environment? The debate is acutely relevant to the biopsychosocial model, which embraces both individualistic and societal perspectives. Attempts to deal with the tension – for example, by noting the *simultaneous* existence of the individual in society and society in the individual (Berger 1963) – simply crystallize the reflexive paradox.

We move next to a discussion of attempts to deal with tangles and loops, in order to see whether there is any hope of rejuvenating the case for an integrated biopsychosocial model in understanding health.

Dealing with reflexive loops

In this section, we assess how different theories and perspectives can deal with reflexive loops or paradoxes. We explore the practice implications of taking alternative approaches to reflexive loops. After considering the theory of logical types, we go on to look at more creative approaches to paradoxes, in order to assess whether any possibility exists of a fully integrated biopsychosocial model being developed.

The Theory of Logical Types was developed by the philosopher Bertrand Russell as a means of dealing with the paradox of reflexive loops by prohibiting them (Whitehead and Russell 1926). Russell argued that a class cannot be a member of itself: 'An element within a context must not loop back upon itself' (Cronen *et al.* 1982: 93). Russell's preoccupation with abolishing reflexivity was related to his broader philosophical position. He believed that the role of language is to represent the world 'out there' in a way that does not lead to confusion. The supposition is that there is an 'untangled', or orderly, reality to make sense of. When reflexive loops are constructed, we can infer that reality is nonsensical, a position that Russell could not tolerate, hence his theory.

Health practitioners may have the same lack of tolerance for reflexivity that Russell expressed. One grass roots solution to paradoxes simply may be to ignore the possibility of one's favoured theory articulating with any other. For example, as Stevenson and Barker suggest in Chapter 4, the professional gets on with what he or she defines as the 'real work', while largely ignoring the activity of other disciplines. The emphasis on one's own perspective excludes reflective practice, which would, in its process, increase the awareness of different theories about health and health care, but would have a negative potential for setting up paradoxical loops and create difficulties in relating to other professionals. What we are contending is that applying Whitehead and Russell's solution is dangerous in practice. A 'head in the sand' approach to other theories mitigates against the biological, psychological and social being *integrated*. A particular world view is taken as correct and immutable. Second, practitioners fail to address power issues, such as those surrounding race, gender, disability and age. For example, suppose a psychiatrist takes the position that a woman's belief about being a member of the royal family is a delusion due to biological disturbance. We are not arguing here that the psychiatrist is either correct or mistaken. However, once a position is taken, the psychiatrist is unlikely to consider the woman's role in relation to her family. Yet an alternative account of her 'delusion', also not given a status as 'right' or 'wrong', is that being royal is a metaphor for the woman's need to assert her position in a traditional male-dominated family organization. Referring specifically to health promotion, Nigel Watson utilized the argument that knowledge and power are inter-linked. When knowledge bases are well rehearsed by the particular professional, lay discourse is a valid way of addressing professional hegemony, of whatever school. Yet the value of lay discourse is unlikely to be acknow-ledged by practitioners who are overly preoccupied with the correctness of their particular explanation.

Whitehead and Russell's (1926) solution to reflexive loops was, by their own definition, interim. More creative solutions to the problem of reflex-ivity have been developed and an exploration of these follows.

In everyday life people do find ways to deal with competing levels of communication, or competing explanations for health phenomena. The ob-jective, as a summary for biological, scientific psychological and positivist sociological explanations of the world, can be defined as a different level of discourse from the subjective, as a summary for social constructionist/ interpretive social psychology and sociology (Hofstadter 1979). However, Hofstadter argued that the two levels are reconcilable. In verbal explana-tions, taking Whitehead and Russell's (1926) position, it can be argued that the reason why different levels of communication, or explanations of health phenomena, are *seen* as irreconcilable is that there is simply no language available with which to describe, or account for, the reflexive loops.

Another way to think about competing theories is in terms of clashing grammars. Grammar is defined as culture-dependent patterns of practice for putting words together. For example, the grammar of biology is patterned by the community of biologists needing to clarify the world through reduc-tion to anatomy, physiology, and so on. Conversely, social constructionist grammatical patterns are a reflection of the complexity of the social world. For example, one way biologists use the term 'mapping' is when represent-ing a gene on the chromosome 'map'. The gene is either present or absent. The map is taken as the exact representation of the territory. For the social constructionist, such a representation is impossible. For example, Cronen *et al.* (1982) took the view that language, or communication, is best not des-cribed as representing or picturing reality. The map is *never* the territory (Hunsley 1993), simply a helpful guide. For social constructionists, com-munication is the process by which people *create* accounts that help them to make sense of their world. For example, when people are faced with a difficult form of communication (e.g. reflexive loops), they construct a narrative, or story, which helps them to deal with it. One possible narrative concerning 'Cretans and lying' is that Epimenedes was teasing when he said that all Cretans are liars. The point is returned to below when the idea that language emerges from practice is explored. That is, one account that could emerge would be about an integrated biopsychosocial model of health and illness.

To explore the potential power of language further, we next undertake an exploration of social constructionism in relation to the biopsychosocial model. We evaluate an alternative position, co-constructivism, which may mediate between social constructionist and reality-driven positions.

Social constructionism, co-constructivism and the biopsychosocial model

Social constructionism rejects the idea that language is a means of depicting a real world of objects. Rather, constructionists conceptualize the world as being created through formative patterns of social interaction. Pearce eloquently states the case:

> Constructionists delight in repudiating cherished virtues of 'mainstream' ways of dealing with social life. We not only abandon the task of 'representing the world' in our theories but claim that such a representation is in principle impossible and in practice pernicious. We construct theories which deliberately eschew a 'foundation' upon which certainty can be grounded on clear, distinct ideas (Rorty 1979; 1989). We forfeit the illusion of certainty in our theories and the dream of reality in our lives (Watzlawick 1976; Segal 1986).
>
> (Pearce 1992: 140)

Thus far, social constructionism has not offered a means of truly integrating different perspectives on health. It steps outside existing positions and seeks to explain how multiple accounts of the world are produced and sustained. In so doing, it deconstructs their hierarchical arrangement. A positive ramification of the deconstruction is that lay beliefs have equal status with those of professionals. There is a potential, when all explanations have equal status, for constructing new accounts. In Chapter 4, Stevenson and Barker comment that professionals may co-create very sophisticated working agreements. However, there are several drawbacks to a social constructionist analysis.

A spirit of tolerance for the explanations, or accounts, offered by others, is based on the recognition that there are many potential realities. Through their tolerance, social constructionist analyses allow expansion in the set of possible explanations for any phenomenon (expansionism). Paradoxically in the context of the present work, removing the hierarchy – by accepting that each explanation is equally valid – takes away the necessity to have any form of integration. This may not necessarily be seen as problematic. From a social constructionist perspective, it is naive to expect that any *one* theory can help us to account for the complex phenomena in health and health care. There is the need for a theoretical ecology (Adams 1990, in Stainton Rogers 1991) in which each theory implicates, but simultaneously excludes, the others. Each account is equally good. Watzlawick (1984) has noted that we live within multiple realities. For example, we note that a glass can be alternatively described as half empty or half full. *Integrating* theories would not enrich the ecology of ideas, or theories, or explanations.

Yet if each account of the world is seen as equally valid as any other, the proliferation of accounts leads to relativism. As Stevenson and Cooper note in Chapter 10, a similar problem arises in selecting a research methodology, in terms of justifying the choice of a particular approach. People have to make choices as they live in the world. If all accounts are equally valid, how do we ever make selections?

Speed (1991) has tried to reconcile the vagaries of positivist approaches (here we refer to reductionist biological and psychological positions and social structural approaches) and the potential relativism of a social constructionist position. She called the new framework co-constructivism. According to Forster and Stevenson in Chapter 11, neither introductionism (as a form of expansionism, or social constructionism) *nor* reductionism (as a form of positivism) are helpful. Speed's solution appears sophisticated enough to deal with relativism without sterilizing the ecology of ideas that multiple accounts allow.

Speed (1991) argued that it is impossible to ignore the physical world, but that there is still room to construct different versions of it. For example, she noted that Family X is physically different from Family Y, but that, although the difference in structure will delimit the range of interpretations of their behaviour, the physical reality will not entirely proscribe the interpretation.

Applying a co-constructivist analysis to the biopsychosocial model, it would be accepted that the person defined as sick has a physical basis to his or her 'sickness'. However, the meanings that are attached to that sickness would be seen to arise through the activity of key 'players' (e.g. the sick person him or herself, the other family members, the professionals). The personhood of the sick person is constructed, or defined, within the limits of the physical world.

A co-constructivist analysis suggests that the physical world sets a context in which health or sickness are defined. It is not a hierarchical analysis, in the sense that we have defined above, because co-constructivism does not have any reductionism or expansionism within it. Rather, any explanation is defined as partial and particular, set within a physical context. Yet within a co-constructivist analysis, there is no extended consideration of the kinds of contextual settings which might be important. We turn next, therefore, to a more detailed analysis of context in frankly hierarchical systems.

The potential for 'integrating' through non-problematic reflexive loops: re-instituting holism

We do not advocate integration of the different parts of the biopsychosocial model, believing that integration would not, in any case, allow us to arrive at an holistic model. In addition, homogenizing the model would delimit the ecology of explanations, a point made earlier in the chapter. Our position is that a more sophisticated means of coordinating the biological, psychological and the social is possible. We begin by establishing that wholes cannot be successfully represented within their parts, and advocate an holistic framework, as defined in Chapter 11. We acknowledge that adding an holistic view of health and illness, alongside biopsychosocial levels, forms a hierarchy which, at first sight, sets up a reflexive paradox as pernicious as those set up by attempts to produce an 'integrated' biopsychosocial model. In referring to such hierarchical systems, Pearce (1992), drawing from the work of (Potter and Wetherall 1987), argued that we are inevitably twisted into a reflexive loop as the perspective from which we describe systems of intelligibility is itself a system of intelligibility. However, a non-problematic reflexive loop can be established. Holism, as defined within this book, can be treated as a context that leads to less problematic reflexive loops.

Lao-Tse expressed the problem of separating parts and whole in the first chapter of the *Tao Te Ching*: 'The Tao that can be expressed is not the real Tao: the name that can be named is not the real name'. As argued by Forster and Stevenson in Chapter 11, a biopsychosocial model reduces the person to constituent parts. Each of the parts is treated by particular professionals as, what Wittgenstein (1953, para. 197) labelled, a 'fixed language game'. In a fixed language game, the rules of the game are re-constituted in playing the game. For example, the medic who asks the patient, 'What are you suffering from?', may invite a response in terms of symptomatology because there is a well-rehearsed grammar in our culture for how to 'go on' from an enquiry about suffering.

A biopsychosocial model is not holistic in the sense that the model does not encompass personhood. Personhood is the totality of a person's being, embedded in his or her social world. One way to think about holism and the biopsychosocial model is that personhood is an emergent property from biopsychosocial levels of functioning. New properties emerge at a higher level of organization of phenomena that are not derivable from the properties of the lower level constituent parts. Because personhood is emergent, it cannot be represented in the parts, a further point made by Forster and Stevenson in Chapter 11.

We have taken time to establish that parts and whole seem to be hier-archically arranged. However, in contrast to the reflexive loops which we have suggested are *necessarily* set up within the biopsychosocial model, we think that holism can provide a 'special' context because it is a concept rather than an explanation. Its specialness means that paradoxes do not necessarily arise, and we return to this point below. However, we want first to establish the characteristics of unproblematic and problematic reflexive loops.

Defining problematic and non-problematic reflexive loops

Cronen *et al.* (1982) noted the need for four processes in order to help us differentiate between problematic and non-problematic loops:

(a) . . . a set of symbols for representing the organisation of social meanings. The symbols (after Cronen *et al.* 1982: 100), arranged in order of their contextual weight are:
Cultural patterns   Broad patterns of social order and humankind's relationship to that order. These patterns locate human experience in a larger context and legitimise ways of knowing and ways of acting.
Life scripts   The repertories of action that make up a person's concept of self.
Relationship   Understandings, usually implicit, that make up the collective 'we'. Relationship meanings in this system are definitions of the collective 'we'.
Episodes   Communication routines that persons view as wholes. Episodes are comprised of reciprocated speech acts.
Speech acts   The things people do to each other with words or actions. Examples of speech acts are threats, promises, rejection, giving information etc.
Content   Information about anything that is communicable con-taining no indication of what kind of message it is.
In the 'Coordinated Management of Meaning' (Cronen and Pearce 1978) it is argued that the symbols for representing the organisation of social meaning are hierarchically organised, with cultural patterns being the highest symbol and content the lowest.
(b) . . . the concept of transivity which simply refers to whether one social perception can reasonably be the context for another perception.
(c) . . . the concept of metarules. The rules which define *which* social perceptions can be the context of which others.
(d) . . . the information specifying how two levels of social perception may be related to each other is contained in higher-level construc-tions of social organisation and personal experience.

According to Cronen and Pearce (1978: 101) the 'levels of meaning are *integrated* [our emphasis] by constitutive rules that show how meaning at one level of abstraction counts as meaning at another level in light of a context higher than both'. Their assertion is critical to our version of 'integration' of the biopsychosocial model, which sets holism as a higher level conceptual context that can help us to articulate together the meanings that are attached to the biological, psychological and social, as argued below.

First, however, in order to understand fully how non-problematic reflexive loops can occur, it is useful to determine what makes the loop problematic? Let us suppose that the relationship which sets the context for the episode does not have a pre-packaged definition (e.g. as a head-to-head relationship or a collaborative relationship). In other words, the relationship emerges *alongside* episodes. If the emergent relationship is consistent with the episodes that take place, the pairing is 'transitive' and not problematic. For example, a collaborative relationship and episode of mutually empathic discussion about the difficulty of an area of professional practice are not in conflict. If the episode and relationship are not consistent, then the problematic loop is set up. For example, take a collaborative relationship which arises between two professionals. An explanatory episode in which one person asserts that 'biology is important', and the other person that 'psychology is important', could be read by each person as an attempt to work together to ensure that all aspects of care are given, *or* as a challenge to her own ideas. The reading depends on which level of meaning is prioritized, the episode itself or the relationship. There is a strange loop, because each person is unclear about how to assign meaning to an experience. The joining of the relationship and episode is intransitive. The consequence of the person recognizing a strange loop is an effect on their behaviour. For example, should the receiver of the message 'biology is important', in response to her assertion about psychology, respond with 'yes, we are in agreement about that', or reiterate the importance of psychology (e.g. 'it's not as important as psychology'). Having identified how problematic loops occur, what responses can be made which allow a different outcome?

Cronen *et al.* (1982) suggested that a helpful response is to define metarules. These are ways of defining which social perceptions (or explanations) can be the context of which others. Let us begin to set out the metarules that draw on holism as a high-level context for 'integrating' the biopsychosocial levels of explanation. First, however, we will remind the reader of our previous position on the biopsychosocial model and holism.

We have claimed that the biopsychosocial model is a hierarchically arranged system of explanations. We considered that this biopsychosocial system and holism can also be seen as hierarchically arranged. A problem might arise if we claim holism (as personhood) as both a larger context for, *and* as integral to, the biopsychosocial model (i.e. claiming to have a theory of personhood within each level of explanation). However, we like Cronen and co-workers' (1982) idea of contextual influence. Context, as used here, is more than a static 'backdrop'. It is an activity through which a potentially new meaning framework is woven together, from which existing under-standings are seen in a 'new light'. A high-level contextual force can exert a force downwards and prevent reflexive loops between two lower levels being established. Thus, an holistic model of care, one which respects per-sonhood as something beyond the sum of the constituent biological, psycho-logical and social parts, can set a high-level context in which the meanings attached to the biological, psychological and social individually can be accounted for in terms of the meanings they have for each other, because of the provision of metarules. The following example illustrates the point.

Suppose a community psychiatric nurse (CPN) is provided with a ready-made 'script' about holism as personhood through reading a professional journal, or this book. The script can be described as an holistic, humanistic cultural programme, or high-level context for CPN work. Holism, as a cultural context, will include beliefs, rituals, customs and conventions. As Hannah (1994: 70) suggested, 'I describe culture as a context in which we create "rules" for living in coordination with others, thereby knowing how to act in given situations'. The cultural context will not be static, but will evolve through the action of its members. It will have both stability and flexibility and evolutionary openness. As such, holism may be seen as what Wittgenstein (cited in Baker and Hacker 1985: 91) called a 'centre of varia-tion'. It sets a framework in which practice can take place with creativity, while remaining consistent with past use, through the perception of what Wittgenstein called 'family resemblances' rather than through the identi-fication of an holistic essence. Against an holistic 'backdrop', the prac-titioner's accounts of his or her practice might consist of constructions of social organization and personal experience which contain information about how two levels of social perception (levels of explanation) may be related to each other. For example, the CPN may continue to consider how biological changes associated with medication are physically dangerous, but also introduce the metarule that biological changes have a meaning at the psychological level, in terms of self-image, because self-image is relevant to personhood.

How might such metarules arise in practice? Practitioners of different disciplinary allegiances, as Stevenson and Barker argue in Chapter 4, some-how do work together in their everyday practice. Cronen and Lang (1994) suggested that helping professionals are practitioners of an art. The practice (or praxis) is living in and by communication and conversation. They do not make a firm distinction between theory and practice. We suggest that ac-counts which practitioners give of how they function together, in terms of their differing explanations, are 'practical theories', in Cronen and Lang's (1994) terms. Practitioners might weave a web of interconnecting stories derived from different levels of context (e.g. an holistic culture and an interdisciplinary episode), thereby providing a coherence in how to act with other practitioners. In connecting stories together, each party is grasping the rules for the other's practice in a way that helps the other to respond so that *both* parties can 'go on' coherently. It is an emergent rules language game where the practitioners create and re-create the grammar which allows them to 'carry on practising'. 'Entailed in this emergent grammar is a different "lived experience" and different forms of relating . . .' (Cronen and Lang 1994: 27). Pearson notes in Chapter 2 how the integration of different explanations occurred *in practice*, as new understandings emerged which allowed each professional to respond in a more positive way to the other's world view. Practitioners live the stories they tell about the reflexive loop. In turn, the stories told are modified through the process of living.

Cronen and Lang (1994) pointed out that telling stories about lived episodes is a learned ability; for example, a child may begin by telling a story from the middle and this is not immediately comprehensible to the adult listener because it does not follow a description of the preceding events. Health professionals may live stories as coordinated practice but have yet to learn to tell the stories about that practice, in order to open up the conversational domain. Developing stories about holistic, coordinated practice must inevitably mean that practice will be affected as those stories are lived. New stories will, in turn, emerge as older stories are lived, which will enhance the cultural context of holism. As Cronen and Lang (1994: 6) stated, 'People do not merely exchange messages or become coupled by communication. Rather, such practitioners "act into" the actions of the other and in so doing create who they are, their social abilities and a social world'.

Conclusion

The chapter has reviewed the complexity of producing a reconciling framework in relation to biological, psychological and sociological explanations. These are different forms of explanation. Different explanations of health phenomena are described as hierarchically arranged. Those forms of explanation which are non-intentional (e.g. biological or social structural) are often seen as superior.

The hierarchical arrangement leads to tangles of meaning, or reflexive loops or paradoxes. The tension between the individual and the social indicates a reflexive paradox – individual in society *and* society in the individual? There have been diverse suggestions as to how to deal with paradoxical, reflexive loops. Rules to ban reflexivity (e.g. by disallowing the source of confusion) are not helpful. Similarly, when practitioners take a singular perspective, lay explanations, power and gender issues may be ignored.

Different solutions to reflexivity among levels of explanation have been proposed. For example, it has been suggested that an integrated biopsychosocial model could be socially constructed through discourse. However, social constructionists mainly have deconstructed existing ways of knowing our world, rather than providing an alternative epistemology. They see different accounts of the world as equally valid, and a rich ecology of ideas results. But the expansion of possibilities leads to problems of relativism. Co-constructivism offers an antidote to relativism, as the reality of a world 'out there' is accepted. However, it does not incorporate a sophisticated analysis of the place of context.

An analysis of reflexive loops suggests a means of integrating levels of the biopsychosocial model in the context of holism as 'personhood'. Holism can be the impetus for developing metarules about the coordination of different levels of explanation.

References

Abbott, P. and Wallace, C. (1990) Social work and nursing: A history, in P. Abbott and C. Wallace (eds) *The Sociology of the Caring Professions*. Basingstoke: Falmer Press.

Adams, L. (1994) Health promotion in crisis, *Health Education Journal*, 53: 353–60.

Adams, L. and Smithies, J. (1990) *Community Participation and Health Promotion*. London: Health Education Authority.

Adams, R. (1990) *Self Help, Social Work and Empowerment*. London: Macmillan.

Aggleton, P. (1990) *Health*. London: Routledge and Kegan Paul.

Aggleton, P. and Chalmers, H. (1986) *Nursing Models and the Nursing Process*. Basingstoke: Macmillan Education.

Aggleton, P. and Chalmers, H. (1987) Models of nursing, nursing practice and nurse education, *Journal of Advanced Nursing*, 12: 573–81.

Allen-Meares, P. and Lane, B.A. (1990) Social work practice: Integrating qualitative and quantitative data collection techniques, *Social Work*, 35: 452–6.

Anderson, H. and Goolishian, H. (1992) The client is the expert: A not-knowing approach to therapy. In S. McNamee and K.J. Gergen (eds). *Therapy as Social Construction*. London: Sage.

Archer, J. and Rhodes, V. (1987) Bereavement and reactions to job loss: A comparative review, *British Journal of Social Psychology*, 26: 211–24.

Armstrong, D. (1983) *The Political Anatomy of the Body*. Cambridge: Cambridge University Press.

Ashton, J. and Seymour, H. (1988) *The New Public Health: The Liverpool Experience*. Milton Keynes: Open University Press.

Atkin, K., Lunt, N., Parker, G. and Hirst, M. (1993) *Nurses Count – A National Census of Practice Nurses*. York: Social Policy Research Unit, University of York.

Atkinson, B.J., Heath, A.W. and Chenail, R. (1991) Qualitative research and the legitimisation of knowledge, *Journal of Marital and Family Therapy, 17*: 175–80.

Backett, K. (1992) The construction of health knowledge in middle class families, *Health Education Research, 7*: 497–507.

Bagenal, F.S., Easton, D.F. and Harris, E. (1990) The survival of patients with breast cancer attending the Bristol Cancer Help Centre, *Lancet, 336*: 606–10.

Baistow, K. (1994/95) Liberation and regulation? Some paradoxes of empowerment, *Critical Social Policy, 14*: 34–46.

Baker, G.P. and Hacker, P.M.S. (1985) *Essays on the Philosophical Investigations: Vol. 1. Wittgenstein: Meaning and Understanding.* Chicago, IL: University of Chicago Press.

Barnardos (1995) *Changing Childhood.* Basingstoke: Barnardos Publishing.

Bateson, G. (1972) *Steps to an Ecology of Mind.* New York: Ballantine.

Beard, H. and Cerf, C. (1992) *The Official Politically Correct Dictionary and Handbook.* London: Grafton.

Beattie, A. (1991) Knowledge and control in health promotion: A test case for social policy and social theory, in J. Gabe and D. Kelleher (eds) *The Sociology of the Health Service.* London: Routledge and Kegan Paul.

Beattie, A. (1993) The changing boundaries of health, in A. Beattie, M. Gott, L. Jones and M. Sidell (eds) *Health and Well-being: A Reader.* Basingstoke: Macmillan.

Beck, U. (1992) From industrial society to risk society: Questions of survival, social structure and ecological enlightenment, *Theory Culture and Society, 9*: 97–123.

Belsey, M.A. (1993) Child abuse: measuring a global problem. *World Health Statistics Quarterly, 46*: 69–77.

Belsky, J. (1980) Child maltreatment: An ecological integration, *American Psychologist, 35*: 320–35.

Bendall, E. (1975) *So You Passed Nurse?* London: Royal College of Nursing.

Benner, P. (1984) *From Novice to Expert.* Menlo Park, CA: Addison-Wesley.

Benner, P. and Wrubel, J. (1989) *The Primacy of Caring: Stress and Coping in Health and Illness.* Menlo Park, CA: Addison-Wesley.

Berger, P. (1963) *Invitation to Sociology.* Harmondsworth: Penguin.

Berger, P. and Luckmann, T. (1967) *The Social Construction of Reality.* London: Allan Lane.

Berne, E. (1968) *Games People Play.* Harmondsworth: Penguin.

Bernstein, R. (1983) *Beyond Objectivism and Relativism: Science, Hermeneutics and Praxis.* Philadelphia, PA: University of Pennsylvania Press.

Biehal, N. and Sainsbury, E. (1991) From values to rights in social work, *British Journal of Social Work, 21*: 245–57.

Birch, J. (1995) Chasing the rainbow's end, and why it matters: A coda to Frosh, Pocock and Larner, *Journal of Family Therapy, 17*: 219–28.

Biswas, B. (1993) The medicalization of dying: A nurse's view, in D. Clark (ed.) *The Future for Palliative Care: Issues of Policy and Practice.* Buckingham: Open University Press.

Black Report (1980) *Inequalities in Health: Report of a Research Working Group.* London: Department of Health and Social Security.

Blackburn, C. (1993) Gender, class and smoking cessation work, *Health Visitor, 66*: 83–5.

Blaxter, M. (1983) Health services as a defence against the consequences of poverty in industrialized societies. *Social Science and Medicine, 17*: 1139–48.

Blaxter, M. (1990) *Health and Lifestyles*. London: Tavistock/Routledge and Kegan Paul.

Blaxter, M. and Paterson, L. (1982) *Mothers and Daughters*. London: Heinemann.

Bloor, M. and McIntosh, J. (1990) Surveillance and concealment: A comparison of techniques of client resistance in therapeutic communities and health visiting, in S. Cunningham-Burley and N.P. McKeganey (eds) *Readings in Medical Sociology*. London: Routledge and Kegan Paul.

Bordo, S. (1990) Reading the slender body, in M. Jacobus, E. Fox Keller and S. Shuttleworth (eds) *Body/Politics*. London: Routledge and Kegan Paul.

Bornstein, M.H. (1984) Psychology's relations with allied intellectual disciplines: An overview, in M.H. Bornstein (ed.) *Psychology and its Allied Disciplines: Vol. 3. The Natural Sciences*. Hillsdale, NJ: Lawrence Erlbaum Associates.

Boston, S. and Trezise, R. (1988) Merely Mortal: Coping with Dying, Death and Bereavement. London: Methuen.

Bowlby, J. (1961) Processes of mourning, *International Journal of Psychoanalysis, 42*: 317–40.

Bowlby, J. (1980) *Attachment and Loss: Vol. 3. Loss: Sadness and Depression*. Harmondsworth: Penguin.

Bowling, A. (1983) Teamwork in primary health care, *Nursing Times*, 30 November, pp. 56–9.

Boyd, M., Brummell, K., Billingham, K. and Perkins, E. (1993) *The Public Health Post at Strelley: An Interim Report*. Nottingham: Nottingham Community Health NHS Trust.

Brewin, T.B. (1994) Chernobyl and the media, *British Medical Journal, 309*: 208–9.

British Association of Social Workers (1985) *The Management of Child Abuse*. Birmingham: BASW.

British Holistic Medical Association (1986) *Report of the British Medical Association Board of Science Working Party on Alternative Therapies*. London: BHMA.

British Medical Association (1986) *Alternative Therapy*. London: BMA.

Bryman, A. (1988) *Quantity and Quality in Social Research*. London: Unwin Hyman.

Buckeldee, J. (1989) A preliminary analysis of the role and interactions of the district nurse with lay carers in the community. Unpublished MSc thesis, King's College, University of London.

Buckman, R. and Sabbagh, K. (1993) *Magic or Medicine? An Investigation into Healing*. London: Macmillan.

Bunton, R. and Macdonald, G. (eds) (1992) *Health Promotion Disciplines and Diversity*. London: Routledge and Kegan Paul.

Burk, C. and Sikora, K. (1992). Cancer: The dual approach, *Nursing Times, 88*: 62–6.

Caplan, R. and Holland, R. (1990) Rethinking health education theory. *Health Education Journal, 49*: 10–12.

Carr, W. and Kemmis, S. (1986) *Becoming Critical: Education, Knowledge and Action Research*. Basingstoke: Falmer Press.

Carson, V. (1994) Caring: The rediscovery of our nursing roots, *Perspectives in Psychiatric Care, 30*: 4–6.

Cassileth, B.R. (1982) Sounding boards: After Lactril, what?, *New England Journal of Medicine, 306*: 1482–4.

Charlton, B.G. (1993) Holistic medicine or the humane doctor?, *British Journal of General Practice, 43*: 475–7.

Charlton, B., Calvert, N., White, M., Rye, G., Conrad, W. and van Zwanenberg, T. (1994) Health promotion priorities for general practice: Constructing and using 'indicative prevalences', *British Medical Journal, 308*: 1019–22.

Christie, A. (1993) Putting career involvement in child protection into practice, in H. Ferguson, R. Gilligan and R. Torode (eds) *Surviving Childhood Adversity: Issues for Policy and Practice.* Dublin: Social Studies Press.

Clark, J. (1973) *A Family Visitor.* London: Royal College of Nursing.

Cleveland Report (1988) *Report of the Inquiry into Child Abuse in Cleveland 1987.* London: HMSO.

Clifford, C. (1993) The clinical role of the nurse teacher in the United Kingdom, *Journal of Advanced Nursing, 18*: 281–9.

Cloke, C. and Davies, M. (eds) (1995) *Participation and Empowerment in Child Protection.* London: Pitman Press.

Cochran, L. and Claspell, E. (1987) *The Meaning of Grief: A Dramaturgical Approach to Understanding Emotion.* London: Greenwood Press.

Cooper, C.L. (1988) Personality, life stress and cancerous disease, in S. Fisher and J.T. Reason (eds), *Handbook of Life Stress, Cognition and Health.* Chichester: John Wiley.

Cooper, N.J. and Pennington, D.C. (1995) The attitudes of social workers, health visitors and school nurses to parental involvement in child protection case conferences. *British Journal of Social Work, 25*: 599–613.

Corby, B. (1987) Why ignoring the rights of parents in child abuse cases should be avoided, *Social Work Today, 19*: 8–9.

Corby, B. (1989) Alternative theory bases in child abuse, in W. Stainton Rogers, D. Hevey and E. Ash (eds) *Child Abuse and Neglect: Facing the Challenge.* London: Batsford.

Council for the Education and Training of Health Visitors (1977) *An Investigation into the Principles of Health Visiting.* London: Council for the Education and Training of Health Visitors.

Cowley, S. (1994) Skill mix: Value for whom?, *Health Visitor, 66*: 166–8.

Cowley, S. (1995) Health promotion in the general practice setting, *Health Visitor, 68*: 199–201.

Creighton, S.J. (1992) *Child Abuse Trends in England and Wales. 1988–1990.* London: NSPCC.

Cronen, V.E. and Lang, P. (1994) Language and action: Wittgenstein and Dewey in the practice of therapy and consultation, *Human Systems: The Journal of Systemic Consultation and Management, 5*: 5–43.

Cronen, V.E. and Pearce, W.B. (1982) The logic of the coordinated management of meanings: An open systems model of interpersonal communication, cited in V.E. Cronen, K.M. Johnson and J.W. Lannaman, Paradoxes, double binds and reflexive loops: An alternative perspective, *Family Process, 21*: 91–112.

Cronen, V.E., Johnson, K.M. and Lannaman, J.W. (1982) Paradoxes, double binds and reflexive loops: An alternative perspective, *Family Process, 21*: 91–112.

Curnock, K. and Hardiker, P. (1979) *Towards Practice Theory: Skills and Methods in Social Assessment.* London: Routledge and Kegan Paul.

Daly, M. and Wilson, M. (1985) Child abuse and other risks of not living with both parents, *Ethology and Sociobiology, 6*: 197–210.

Decker, T., Cline, E.J. and Gallagher, M. (1992) Relaxation as an adjunct in radiation oncology, *Journal of Clinical Psychology, 48*: 388–93.

De Haes, J.C.J.M., Knippenberg, F.C.E. and Neijt, J.P. (1990) Measuring psychological and physical distress in cancer patients: Structure and application of the Rotterdam symptom checklist, *British Journal of Cancer, 62*: 1034–8.

Delamothe, T. (1991) Social inequalities in health, *British Medical Journal, 303*: 1046–50.

Dennett, D.C. (1984) Computer models and the mind: A view from the east pole, *Times Literary Supplement*, 14 December, p. 1453.

Denton, P. (1992) Make your voice heard (Complementary therapy supplement), *Nursing Standard, 6*: 50.

Department of Health (1989) *The Children's Act*. London: HMSO.

Department of Health (1991a) *The Patients' Charter, El(91)128*. London: Department of Health.

Department of Health (1991b) *Working Together*. London: HMSO.

Department of Health (1992) *The Health of the Nation: A Strategy for Health in England*, Cmnd 1986. London: HMSO.

Department of Health (1993) *Changing Childbirth. Part 1: Report of the Expert Working Group*. London: HMSO.

Department of Health (1994) *The Challenge of Partnership: A Guide for Practitioners*. London: HMSO.

Department of Health and Social Security (1974) Non-accidental injury to children. LASSL (74) 13.

Department of Health and Social Security (1976) *Report of the Committee on Child Health Services: Fit for the Future (The Court Report)*. London: HMSO.

Department of Health and Social Security and the Welsh Office (1987) *AIDS: Monitoring Response to the Public Education Campaign February 1986–February 1987*. London: HMSO.

Department of Health and Social Security and the Welsh Office (1991) *Working Together: A Guide to Arrangements for Inter-agency Co-operation for the Protection of Children from Abuse*. London: HMSO.

Department of Health and the Welsh Office (1989) *General Practice in the National Health Service: A New Contract*. London: DoH and Welsh Office.

Derbyshire County Council (1978) *Report of Professor J.D. McClean concerning Karen Spencer to the Derbyshire County Council and Derbyshire Health Authority*. Derbyshire County Council.

Dingwall, R. (1976) *Aspects of Illness*. London: Martin Robertson.

Dingwall, R. (1986) The Jasmine Beckford affair, *Modern Law Review, 49*: 489–507.

Dingwall, R., Eekelaar, J. and Murray, T. (1983) *The Protection of Children: State Intervention and Family Life*. Oxford: Blackwell.

Dingwall, R., Rafferty, A. and Webster, C. (1988) *An Introduction to the Social History of Nursing*. London: Routledge and Kegan Paul.

Diorio, W.D. (1992) Parental perceptions of the authority of public child welfare caseworkers, *Families in Society, 73*: 222–35.

Doise, W. (1986) *Levels of Explanation in Social Psychology*. Cambridge: Cambridge University Press.

Doll, R. and Peto, R. (1981) *The Causes of Cancer: Quantitative Estimates of Avoidable Risks of Cancer in the US.* Oxford: Oxford University Press.

Douglas, M. (1970) Natural symbols: Explorations in Cosmology. London: Barne and Rockliff, The Cresset Press.

Downie, R.S., Fyfe, C. and Tannahill, A. (1990) *Health Promotion Models and Values.* Oxford: Oxford University Press.

Downie, S.M., Cody, M.M., McCluskey, P., Wilson, P.D., Arnott, S.J., Lister, T.A. and Slevin, M.L. (1994) Pursuit and practice of complementary therapies by cancer patients receiving conventional treatment. *British Medical Journal, 309*: 86–9.

Drennan, V. (1986) A feasibility study into the screening of elderly people in an inner city area, in A. While (ed.) *Research in Preventive Community Nursing Care.* Chichester: John Wiley.

Dunlop, M.J. (1986) Is a science of caring possible?, *Journal of Advanced Nursing, 11*: 661–70.

Dunnell, K. and Dobbs, J. (1983) *Nurses Working in the Community.* London: OPCS/HMSO.

Durkheim, E. (1897/1970) *Suicide: A Study in Sociology.* London: Routledge and Kegan Paul.

Eardley, A. (1986) Patients and radiotherapy: 3. Patients' experience after discharge, *Radiography, 52*: 17–19.

Ehrenreich, B. and English, D. (1973) *Complaints and Disorders: The Sexual Politics of Sickness.* New York: Feminist Press.

Eisenbruch, M. (1984) Cross-cultural aspects of bereavement: A conceptual framework for comparative analysis, *Culture, Medicine and Psychiatry, 8*: 283–309.

Eisner, E.W. (1990) The meaning of alternative paradigms for practice, in E.G. Guba (ed.) *The Paradigm Dialogue.* London: Sage.

Elton-Wilson, J. (1992) Varieties of professional views, *The Psychologist: Bulletin of the British Psychological Society, 5*: 510–12.

Engel, G.L. (1977) The need for a new medical model: A challenge for biomedicine, *Science, 196*: 129–35.

Evans, F. (1987) *The Newcastle Community Midwifery Care Project: An Evaluation Report.* Newcastle: Newcastle Health Authority.

Ewels, L. and Simnett, I. (1985) *Promoting Health – A Practical Guide to Health Education.* Chichester: John Wiley.

Faithfull, S. (1994) The concept of cure in cancer care. *European Journal of Cancer Care, 3*: 12–17.

Falk, P. (1994) *The Consuming Body.* London: Sage.

Fallon, S. (1992) Turning the tide, *Community Care, 908*: 24–6.

Farmer, E. (1993) The impact of child protection interventions, in L. Waterhouse (ed.) *Child Abuse and Child Abusers.* Research Highlights in Social Work Vol. 24. London: Jessica Kingsley.

Farmer, E. and Owen, M. (1995) *Child Protection Practice: Private Risks and Public Remedies.* London: HMSO.

Featherstone, M., Hepworth, M. and Turner, B.S. (eds) (1991) *The Body.* Sage: London.

Felner, R.D., Farber, S.S. and Primavera, J. (1980) Transition and stressful life events: A model for primary prevention, in R. Felner, L. Jason, J. Moritsugu and S.S. Farber (eds) *Preventive Psychology.* New York: Pergamon Press.

Ferguson, K. and Jinks, A.M. (1994) Integrating what is taught with what is practised in the nursing curriculum: A multi-dimensional model, *Journal of Advanced Nursing, 20*: 687–95.

Feyerabend, P. (1991) *Three Dialogues on Knowledge*. Oxford: Basil Blackwell.

Fiore, N. (1979) Fighting cancer: One patient's perspective, *New England Journal of Medicine, 300*: 284–9.

Fiorelli, J.S. (1988) Power in work groups: Team members' perspectives, *Human Relations, 41*: 1–12.

Fisher, R. and Adam, W. (1994) Complementary Medicine in Europe. *British Medical Journal, 309*: 107–11.

Fisher, P. and Ward, A. (1994) Complementary Medicine in Europe, *British Medical Journal, 309*: 107–10.

Fiske, S.T. and Taylor, S.E. (1984) *Social cognition*. Reading MA: Addison-Wesley.

Fissell, M.E. (1991) *The Physic of Charity: Health and Welfare in the West Country 1690–1810*. Cambridge: Cambridge University Press.

Fitch, M. (1992) Integrating research in clinical practice, in C.D. Bailey (ed.) *Cancer Nursing, Changing Frontiers: Proceedings of the Seventh International Conference on Cancer Nursing*, Vienna. Oxford: Rapid Communications of Oxford.

Flaherty, M. (1981) Living with cancer, in R. Tiffany (ed.) *Cancer Nursing Update*. London: Baillière Tindall.

Ford, P. and Walsh, M. (1994) *New Rituals for Old*. London: Heinemann.

Foucault, M. (1963) *Naissance de la Clinique*. Paris: Presses Universitaires de France. English translation (1973) *The Birth of the Clinic*. Tavistock: London.

Foucault, M. (1975) *The Archaeology of Knowledge*. London: Tavistock.

Fowler, G. (1993) The Indians' revenge, *British Journal of General Practice, 43*: 78–81.

Frankel, J. (1990) Parental participation at case conferences: An analysis of the Maidstone Social Services Area 'Pilot Scheme'. Unpublished paper, London, Hedley Library.

Franklin, B. (1989) Children's rights: developments and prospects. *Children and Society, 31*: 76–92.

Freeman, M.D.A. (1983) Freedom and the welfare state: child-rearing, parental autonomy and state intervention. *Journal of Social Welfare Law*, March: 70–91.

French, C. (1984) Competing orientations in child abuse management, *British Journal of Social Work, 14*: 615–24.

Fretwell, J. (1982) *Ward Teaching and Learning*. London: Royal College of Nursing.

Frude, N. (ed.) (1980) *Psychological Approaches to Child Abuse*. London: Becksford.

Frugerri, L. and Matteini, M. (1988) Larger systems? Beyond a dualistic approach to the process of change, *Irish Journal of Psychology, 9*: 183–94.

Fry, A. (1990) There but for the grace, *Social Work Today*, 4 October, p. 16.

Fulder, S. (1988) *Handbook of Complementary Medicine*, 2nd edn. Oxford: Oxford University Press.

Fulder, S.J. and Monro, R. (1981) *The Status of Complementary Medicine in the United Kingdom*. London: Threshold Foundation.

Furnham, A., Pendleton, D. and Manicorn, C. (1981) The perceptions of different occupations within the medical profession, *Social Science and Medicine, 15*: 289–300.

Furniss, T. (1991) *The Multi-professional Handbook of Child Sexual Abuse*. London: Routledge and Kegan Paul.

Gallmeier, T.M. and Bonner, B.L. (1992) University-based interdisciplinary training in child abuse and neglect, *Child Abuse and Neglect, 16*: 513–21.

Gamarnikow, E. (1978) Sexual division of labour: The case of nursing, in A. Kuhn and A. Wolpe (eds) *Feminism and Materialism*. London: Routledge and Kegan Paul.

Garbarino, J. (1977) The human ecology of child maltreatment: A conceptual model for research. *Journal of Marriage and the Family, 39*: 721–35.

Gelfand, T. (1980) *Professionalizing Modern Medicine: Paris Surgeons' Traditional Science and Institutions in the Eighteenth Century*. Westport, CT: Greenwood Press.

George, M. (1992) Conquering cancer, *Nursing Standard, 6*: 22–3.

Gergen, K.J. (1985) The social constructionist movement in modern psychology, *American Psychologist, 40*: 266–75.

Gil, D.G. (1970) *Violence Against Children*. Cambridge, MA: Harvard University Press.

Gil, D.G. (1979) Unravelling child abuse, in D.G. Gil (ed.) *Child Abuse and Violence*. New York: AMS Press.

Gillham, B. (1994) *The Facts About Child Physical Abuse*. London: Cassell.

Glaser, B. G. and Strauss, A.L. (1965) *Awareness of Dying*. Chicago, IL: Aldine.

Glaser, B. G. and Strauss, A.L. (1967) *The Discovery of Grounded Theory: Strategies for Qualitative Research*. Chicago, IL: Grune and Stratton.

Golann, S. (1987) On description of family therapy, *Family Process, 26*: 331–40.

Goodwin, S. (1982) *Whither Health Visiting?* London: Health Visitors' Association.

Gorer, G. (1965) *Death, Grief and Mourning in Contemporary Britain*. London: Cresset Press.

Gould, S.J. (1981) *The Mismeasure of Man*. Harmondsworth: Penguin.

Gould, S.J. (1989) *An Urchin in the Storm*. New York: Norton.

Graham, H. and McKee, L. (1980) *The First Months of Motherhood*, Health Education Council Monograph No. 3. London: Health Education Council.

Green, P. and Kinghorn, S.W. (1994) Radiotherapy: Its nature and scope, in J. David (ed.) *Cancer Care Prevention, Treatment and Palliation*. London: Chapman and Hall.

Greer, S. and Moorey, S. (1987) Adjuvant psychological therapy for patients with cancer, *European Journal of Surgical Oncology, 13*: 511–16.

Guba, E.G. (1990) The alternative paradigm dialog, in E.G. Guba (ed.) *The Paradigm Dialog*. London: Sage.

Guyatt, G., Sackett, D., Adachi, J. and Roberts, R. (1988) A clinician's guide for conducting randomised trials in individual patients, *Canadian Medical Association Journal, 139*: 497–503.

Haley, J. (1963) *Strategies of Psychotherapy*. New York: Grune and Stratton.

Hall, D. (1991) *Health for All Children*. Oxford: Oxford University Press.

Hallett, C. (1993) Working together in child protection, in L. Waterhouse (ed.) *Child Abuse and Child Abusers*. Research Highlights in Social Work Vol. 24. London: Jessica Kingsley.

Hallett, C. and Stevenson, O. (1980) *Child Abuse: Aspects of Interprofessional Co-operation*. London: Allen and Unwin.

Hannah, C. (1994) The context of culture in systemic therapy: An application of CMM, *Human Systems: The Journal of Systemic Consultation and Management,* 5: 69–81.

Hardiker, P. and Barker, M. (eds) (1981) *Theories of Practice in Social Work.* London: Academic Press.

Harré, R. (1971) Joynson's dilemma, *Bulletin of the British Psychological Society,* 24: 115–19.

Harré, R. (1981) The positivist, empiricist approach and its alternative, in P. Reason and J. Rowan (eds) *Human Inquiry.* New York: John Wiley.

Harré, R. (1986) *The Social Construction of Emotion.* Oxford: Blackwell.

Harris, A. (1991) General practitioners and child protection case conferences, *British Medical Journal,* 302: 1354.

Hartman, A. (1970) To think about the unthinkable, *Social Casework,* 51: 467–74.

Hawkins, P. (1989) Reflecting on models of practice. Paper presented at the *Conference of the Sunderland Grief and Loss Centre,* Durham, October.

Health Visitor (1991) Editorial: Wide of the mark, *Health Visitor,* 64: 173.

Health Visitor (1994) Editorial: Gone with the wind?, *Health Visitor,* 67: 325.

Helman, C. (1978) Feed a cold, starve a fever, *Culture, Medicine and Psychiatry,* 2: 107–37.

Hendricks, H. (1990) Constructions and reconstructions of British childhood: An interpretive survey, 1800 to the present, in A.J. James and A. Prout (eds) *Constructing and Reconstructing Childhood: Contemporary Issues in the Sociological Study of Childhood.* Basingstoke: Falmer Press.

Henriques, J., Holloway, W., Urwin, C., Venn, C. and Walkerdine, V. (1984) *Changing the Subject: Psychology, Social Regulation and Subjectivity.* London: Methuen.

Henwood, K.L. and Nicholson, P. (1995) Qualitative research, *The Psychologist: Bulletin of the British Psychological Society,* 8: 109–14.

Henwood, K.L. and Pidgeon, N.J. (1992) Qualitative research and psychological theorising, *British Journal of Psychology,* 83: 97–111.

Hersen, N. and Barlow, D.H. (1976) *Single Case Experimental Designs: Strategies for Studying Behavioural Change.* New York: Pergamon Press.

Hersh, E.S. and Peterson E.A. (1988) Editorial. The AIDS epidemic: AIDS research in the life sciences, *Life Sciences,* 423: i–iv.

Herzberger, S.D. (1988) Cultural obstacles to the labelling of abuse by professionals, in A. Maney and S. Wells (eds) *Professional Responsibilities in Protecting Children: A Public Approach to Child Sexual Abuse.* New York: Praeger.

Hick, J. (1976) On conflicting religious truth claims, *Religious Studies,* 19: 485–91.

Hoagland, A.C. (1983) Bereavement and personal constructs: Old theories and new concepts, *Death Education,* 7: 175–93.

Hobbs, C. and Wynne, J. (1989) Sexual abuse of English boys and girls: The importance of anal examination, *Child Abuse and Neglect,* 13: 195–210.

Hochstadt, N.J. and Harwick, N.J. (1985) How effective is the multi-disciplinary approach? *Child Abuse and Neglect,* 9: 365–72.

Hoffman, L. (1985) Beyond power and control: Towards a second order family systems therapy, *Family Systems Medicine,* 3: 381–96.

Hofstadter, D.R. (1979) *Gödel, Escher, Bach: An Eternal Golden Braid.* Harmondsworth: Penguin.

Hofstadter, D.R. and Dennett, D.C. (1981) *The Mind's I: Fantasies and Reflections on Self and Soul*. Brighton: Harvester.

Howitt, D. (1992) *Child Abuse Errors*. Hemel Hempstead: Harvester Wheatsheaf.

Hunsley, J. (1993) Research and family therapy: Exploring some hidden assumptions, *Journal of Systemic Therapies*, 12: 63–70.

Hunt, J.M. (1974) *The Teaching and Practice of Surgical Dressings in Three Hospitals*. London: Royal College of Nursing.

Iles, P. and Auluck, R. (1990) Team building, interagency team development and social work practice, *British Journal of Social Work*, 20: 151–64.

Illich, I. (1975) *Medical Nemesis – The Expropriation of Health*. London: Calder and Boyars.

Jacobson, B., Smith, A. and Whitehead, M. (1991) *The Nation's Health*, revised edn. London: Health Education Authority.

Janchill, M.P. (1969) Systems concepts in casework theory and practice, *Social Casework*, 50: 74–82.

Jewson, N. (1976) The disappearance of the sick man from medical cosmology, 1770–1870, *Sociology*, 10: 225–44.

Johnson, D.E. (1980) The behavioural systems model for nursing, in J.P. Riehl and C. Roy (eds) *Conceptual Models for Nursing Practice*. New York: Appleton-Century-Crofts.

Johnson, P. (1990) *Child Abuse: Understanding the Problem*. Marlborough: Crowood Press.

Jones, L. (1994) *The Social Context of Health and Health Work*. Basingstoke: Macmillan.

Joynson, R.B. (1971) The breakdown of modern psychology. *Bulletin of the British Psychological Society*, 23: 261–9.

Kabat-Zinn, J. (1994) Foreword, in M. Lerner (ed.) *Choices in Healing*. Cambridge, MA: MIT Press.

Kamerman, J.B. (1988) *Death in the Midst of Life: Social and Cultural Influences on Death, Grief and Mourning*. London: Prentice Hall.

Kane, R.A. (1975) *Inter-professional Teamwork*, Social Work Manpower Monograph No. 8, Syracuse, NY: Syracuse University School of Social Work.

Kaufman, J. and Zigler, E. (1992) The prevention of child maltreatment: Programming, research and policy, in D.J. Willis, E.W. Holden and M. Rosenberg (eds) *Prevention of Child Maltreatment: Developmental and Ecological Perspectives*: New York: Wiley.

Keeney, B.P. (1983) *Aesthetics of Change*. New York: Guilford Press.

Kelly, L. (1992) Outrageous injustice, *Community Care*, 908: ii–iii.

Kempe, C.H., Silverman, F.N., Steele, B.B., Droegemueller, W. and Silver, H.K. (1962) The battered child syndrome, *Journal of the American Medical Association*, 181: 17–24.

Kikuchi, J.F. and Simmons, H. (eds) (1992) *Philosophic Inquiry in Nursing*. London: Sage.

King, L.S. (1982) *Medical Thinking*. Princeton, NJ: Princeton University Press.

Kline, P. (1988) *Psychology Exposed: Or the Emperor's New Clothes*. London: Routledge and Kegan Paul.

Koestler, A. (1964) *The Act of Creation*. New York: Macmillan.

Krippendorf, K. (1991) Reconstructing (some) communication research methods, in F. Steier (ed.) *Research and Reflexivity*. London: Sage.

Kuhn, T.S. (1962) *The Structure of Scientific Revolutions*. Chicago, IL: University of Chicago Press.

La Fontaine, J. (1990) *Child Sexual Abuse*. Cambridge: Polity Press.

Laffan, G. (1993) A new holistic science, *Nursing Standard, 7*: 44–5.

Laing, R.D. (1960) *The Divided Self*. Harmondsworth: Penguin.

Lake, T. (1984) *Living with Grief*. London: Sheldon Press.

Lalonde, M. (1974) *A New Perspective on the Health of Canada*. Ottowa: Information Canada.

Lather, P. (1984) Postmodernism and the politics of enlightenment, *Educational Foundations, 3*: 7–28.

Laurance, A. (1994) *Cancer Concerns*. London. Routledge.

Lawrence, C. (1994) *Medicine in the Making of Modern Britain 1700–1920*. London: Routlege.

Lea-Cox, C. and Hall, A. (1991) Attendance of general practitioners at child protection case conferences, *British Medical Journal, 302*: 1378–9.

Levitt, C. (1990) Sexual abuse of boys: A medical perspective, in M. Hunter (ed.) *The Sexually Abused Male*. Lexington, MA: Lexington Books.

Lewith, G. (1993) *Complementary medicine: new approaches to good practice. An Appraisal of the BMA Report*. Complementary Therapy in Medicine, 1: 218–20.

Lincoln, Y.S. and Guba, E.G. (1985) *Naturalistic Inquiry*. London: Sage.

Lindemann, E. (1944) Symptomatology and management of acute grief, *American Journal of Psychiatry, 101*: 141–8.

Lindley, P. and Bromley, D. (1995) Continuing professional development, *The Psychologist: Bulletin of the British Psychological Society, 8*: 215–18.

Lister, P. (1987) The misunderstood model, *Nursing Times, 83*: 40–42.

Lloyd, A. (1992) Rebuilding the centre. *Nursing Times, 88*: 16–17.

Locker, D. (1991) Prevention and health promotion, in G. Scrambler (ed.) *Sociology as Applied to Medicine*. London: Baillière-Tindall.

Lofland, L.H. (1985) The social shaping of emotion: The case of grief, *Symbolic Interaction, 8*: 171–90.

London Borough of Brent (1985) *A Child in Trust. The Report of the Panel of Inquiry into the Circumstances surrounding the Death of Jasmine Beckford*. London Borough of Brent.

Loney, M. (1989) Child abuse in a social context, in W. Stainton Rogers, D. Hevey and E. Ash (eds) *Child Abuse and Neglect: Facing the Challenge*. London: Batsford.

Luker, K. (1982) *Evaluating Health Visiting Practice*. London: Royal College of Nursing.

Lupton, D. (1994) *Medicine as Culture*. London: Sage.

Macleod Clark, J. (1993) *From Sick Nursing to Health Nursing: Evolution or Revolution?*, in J. Wilson-Barnett and J. Macleod Clark (eds) *Research in Health Promotion and Nursing*. Basingstoke: Macmillan.

Martin, E. (1987) *The Woman in the Body*. Milton Keynes: Open University Press.

Maturana, H.R. and Varela, F.J. (1980) *Autopoiesis and Cognition: The Realisation of the Living*. Dordrecht: Reidel.

McCormick, J.S. (1979) *The Doctor: Father Figure or Plumber*. Beckenham: Croom Helm.

McEwan, R.T., Davison, N., Forster, D.P., Pearson, P. and Stirling, E. (1990) Screening elderly people in primary care: A randomised controlled trial, *British Journal of General Practice, 40*: 94–7.

McGloin, P. and Turnbull, A. (1987) Strengthening good practice by bringing in the parents. *Social Work Today*, 118(46) 14–16.

McGrath, M. (1991) *Multi-disciplinary Teamwork*. London: Gower.

McIntosh, J. and Dingwall, R. (1978) Teamwork in theory and practice, in R. Dingwall and J. McIntosh (eds) *Readings in the Sociology of Nursing*. London: Churchill Livingston.

McKeown, T. (1976) *The Modern Rise of Population*. Edward Arnold: London.

McLeod, R.S., Taylor, D.W., Cohen, Z. and Cullen, J.B. (1986) Single patient randomised clinical trial, *Lancet, 1*: 726–8.

McWhinney, I.R., Bass, M.J. and Donner, A. (1994) Evaluation of palliative care services, *British Medical Journal, 309*: 1340–42.

Menzies, I.E. (1970) *The Functioning of Social Systems as a Defence Against Anxiety*. London: Tavistock.

Meyer, C. (1976) *Social Work Practice*. New York: Free Press.

Middleton, W., Harris, P. and Hollely, C. (1994) Condom use by heterosexual students: Justifications for unprotected intercourse, *Health Education Journal, 53*: 147–54.

Middleton, W., Raphale, B., Martinek, N. and Misso, V. (1993) Pathological grief reactions, in M.S. Stroebe, W. Stroebe and R.O. Hansson (eds) *Handbook of Bereavement Research and Intervention*. Cambridge: Cambridge University Press.

Miller, A. (1985) The relationship between nursing theory and nursing practice, *Journal of Advanced Nursing, 10*: 417–24.

Monk, D. (1986) Participation not persecution, *Community Care, 635*: 22–3.

Montgomery, S. (1982) Problems in the perinatal prediction of child abuse, *British Journal of Social Work, 12*: 189–96.

Moore, J.G. (1985) *The ABC of Child Abuse Work*. Aldershot: Gower.

Moon, S.M., Dillon, D.R. and Sprenkle, D.H. (1991) On balance and synergy: Family therapy and qualitative research revisited, *Journal of Marital and Family Therapy, 2*: 187–92.

Morgan, D. and Scott, S. (1993) Bodies in a social landscape, in S. Scott and D. Morgan (eds) *Body Matters*. London: Falmer Press.

Morgan, M., Calnan, M. and Manning, N. (1985) *Sociological Approaches to Health and Medicine*. Beckenham: Croom Helm.

Morrison, I. and Smith, R. (1994) The future of medicine, *British Medical Journal, 309*: 1099–100.

Morrison, J., Roberts, J. and Will, D. (1987) Twenty Myths that 'justify' not tackling child sexual abuse. *Social Work Today*. July 20th, 9–11.

Morrison, T., Blackey, C., Butler, A., Fallon, S. and Leith, A. (1990) *Child and Parental Participation in Case Conferences*. Occasional Paper No. 8. London: National Society for the Prevention of Cruelty to Children.

Myers, J.E.B. (1993) Expert testimony regarding child sexual abuse, *Child Abuse and Neglect, 17*: 175–85.

Naidoo, J. (1986) Limits to individualism, in S. Rodmell and A. Watt (eds) *The Politics of Health Education*. London: Routledge and Kegan Paul.

Newell, R. (1992) The single case experimental design: A quantitative method for everyday use, *Nursing Practice, 6*: 24–8.

NHS Management Executive (1993) *FHSL (93) 25 GP Contract Health Promotion Package: Amendments to the Statement of Fees and Allowances.* London: Department of Health.

Nursing Times (1994) Editorial, *Nursing Times, 90*: 5.

Ogier, M. (1986) An ideal sister seven years on, *Nursing Times Occasional Papers, 82*: 54–7.

Oldfield, V. (1992) A healing touch, *Nursing Standard, 6*: 21.

Orem, D. (1971) *Nursing: Concepts of Practice.* New York: McGraw Hill.

Orkney Report (1992) *The Report of the Inquiry into the Removal of Children from Orkney in February 1991* (chaired by Lord Clyde). Edinburgh: HMSO.

Orr, J. (1985) Health visiting and the community, in K. Luker and J. Orr (eds) *Health Visiting.* Oxford: Blackwell.

Orr, J. (1986) Working with women's health groups: The community health movement, in A. White (ed.) *Research in Preventive Community Nursing: Fifteen Studies in Health Visiting.* Chichester: John Wiley.

Orton, H. (1981) *Ward Learning Climate.* London: Royal College of Nursing.

O'Sullivan, J. (1990) Children in the shadow of doubt, *The Independent*, 9 October.

Parkes, C.M. (1972) *Bereavement: Studies of Grief in Adult Life.* Harmondsworth: Penguin.

Parsons, T. (1951) *Toward a General Theory of Action.* London: John Wiley.

Parton, N. (1981) Child abuse, social anxiety and welfare, *British Journal of Social Work, 11*: 391–414.

Parton, N. (1985) *The Politics of Child Protection.* London: Macmillan.

Paterson, J.G. (1992) The importance of teamwork, *International Journal for the Advancement of Counselling, 15*: 289–95.

Payne, C. and Scott, T. (1990) *Developing Supervision of Teams in Field and Residential Social Work.* Paper no.12. London: National Institute of Social Work.

Peace, G. (1991) *Child Sexual Abuse: Professional and Personal Perspectives – Part 2: Interprofessional Collaboration.* Cheadle, Cheshire: Boys and Girls Welfare Society.

Pearce, W.B. (1992) A 'camper's guide' to constructionisms, *Human Systems, 3*: 139–62.

Pearson, P. (1988a) Clients' perceptions of health visiting in the context of their identified health needs: An examination of process. Unpublished PhD thesis, University of Northumbria.

Pearson, P. (1988b) Riverside child health project, in V. Drennan (ed.) *Health Visitors and Groups: Politics and Practice.* London: Heinemann.

Pearson, P. (1995a) Client views of health visiting, in R. Heyman (ed.) *Research in Community Health Care.* London: Chapman and Hall.

Pearson, P. (1995b) Interagency working – reflecting on practice. Paper presented at the *Royal College of Nursing Research Advisory Group Conference*, Belfast, April.

Pearson, P. and Jones, K. (1994) The primary health care non-team, *British Medical Journal, 309*: 1387–8.

Pelton, L. (1978) Child abuse and neglect: The myth of classlessness, *American Journal of Orthopsychiatry, 48*: 608–17.

Pelton, L. (1989) *For Reasons of Poverty: A Critical Analysis of the Public Child Welfare System in the United States.* New York: Praeger.

Pender, N., Walker, S., Frank-Stromborg, M. and Sechrist, K. (1990) *Health Promotion in the Workplace: Making a Difference.* Dekalb, IL: Northern Illinois University.

Perrin, L.A. (1978) *Current Controversies and Issues in Personality.* New York: Wiley.

Pfohl, J. (1976) The 'discovery' of child abuse, *Social Problems*, 24: 310–23.

Phillips, K.C. (1988) Strategies against AIDS, *The Psychologist: Bulletin of the British Psychological Society*, 1: 46–7.

Phillips, K.C. (1989) The psychology of AIDS, in A. Colman and J.G. Beaumont (eds) *Psychology Survey No. 7.* Leicester: British Psychological Society.

Pierret, J. (1993) Constructing discourses about health and their social determinants, in A. Radley (ed.) *Worlds of Illness.* London: Routledge and Kegan Paul.

Pinnell, P. (1988) How do cancer patients express their points of view?, *Sociology of Health and Illness*, 9: 25–45.

Potter, J. and Wetherall, M. (1987) *Discourse and Social Psychology: Beyond Attitudes and Behaviour.* London: Sage.

Poulton, K. (1984) A measure of independence, *Nursing Times*, 22 August, pp. 32–5.

Press, I. (1980) Problems in the definition and classification of medical systems, *Social Science and Medicine*, 14: 45–57.

Priestman, T.J. (1989) *Cancer Chemotherapy: An Introduction*, 3rd edn. London: Springer-Verlag.

Rabin, P.L. and Pate, J.K. (1981) Acute grief, *Southern Medical Journal*, 74: 1468–70.

Radley, A. (1994) *Making Sense of Illness.* London: Sage.

Reason, P. (1988) Whole person medical practice, in P. Reason (ed.) *Human Inquiry in Action: Developments in New Paradigm Research.* London: Sage.

Reason, P. (ed.) (1994) *Participation in Human Inquiry.* London: Sage.

Reason, P. and Rowan, J. (eds) (1981) *Human Inquiry: A Sourcebook of New Paradigm Research.* New York: John Wiley.

Research Unit in Health and Behavioural Change (1989) *Changing the Public Health.* London: John Wiley.

Reynolds, W. (1990) Teaching psychiatric and mental health nursing: A teaching perspective, in W. Reynolds and D. Cormack (eds) *Psychiatric and Mental Health Nursing.* London: Chapman and Hall.

Rhodes, M. (1986) *Ethical Dilemmas in Social Work Practice.* Milwaukee, WI: Family Services America.

Riehl, J. and Roy, C. (eds) (1980) *Conceptual Models for Nursing Practice.* New York: Appleton-Century Crofts.

Rodmell, S. and Watt, A. (1986) *The Politics of Health Education.* London: Routledge and Kegan Paul.

Rogers, M.E. (1970) *An Introduction to the Theoretical Basis of Nursing.* Philadelphia, PA: F.A. Davis.

Roper, N., Logan, W.W. and Tierney, A.J. (1980) *The Elements of Nursing.* Edinburgh: Churchill Livingstone.

Rorty, R. (1979) *Philosophy and the Mirror of Nature.* Princeton, NJ: Princeton University Press.

Rorty, R. (1982) *Consequences of Pragmatism*. Minneapolis, MN: University of Minnesota Press.

Rorty, R. (1989) *Contingency, Irony and Solidarity*. Cambridge: Cambridge University Press.

Rose, N. (1985) *The Psychological Complex*. London: Routledge and Kegan Paul.

Ross, F., Bower, P. and Sibbald, B. (1994) Practice nurses: Characteristics, workload and training needs, *British Journal of General Practice, 44*: 15–18.

Roy, C. (1976) *Introduction to Nursing: An Adaptation Model*. Englewood Cliffs, NJ: Prentice Hall.

Saks, M. (1992) Introduction, in M. Saks (ed.) *Alternative Medicine in Britain*. Oxford: Clarendon Press.

Saltonstall, R. (1993) Healthy bodies, social bodies: Men's and women's concepts and practices of health in everyday life, *Social Science and Medicine, 36*: 7–14.

Salvage, J. (1990) The theory and practice of the new nursing, *Nursing Times, 86*: 42–5.

Sarafino, E.P. (1990) *Health Psychology: Biopsychosocial Interactions*. New York: John Wiley.

Saunders, C. (1977) Dying they live: St Christopher's hospice, in H. Feifel (ed.) *New Meanings of Death*. New York: McGraw-Hill.

Scaife, J. (1993) *Hierarchy and Heterarchy in Systemic Therapy: Reflexivity in Therapy and Consultation*, Year 2 Dissertation, Diploma in Systemic Therapy. Birmingham: University of Birmingham and Charles Burns Unit.

Schön, D.A. (1987) *Educating the Reflexive Practitioner*. San Francisco, CA: Jossey-Bass.

Scott, D.W., Donahue, D.C., Mastrovito, R.C. and Hakes, T.B. (1986) Comparative trial of clinical relaxation and an anti-emetic drug regimen in reducing chemotherapy related nausea and vomiting, *Cancer Nursing, 9*: 178–87.

Seebohm Committee (1968) *Report of the Committee on Local Authority and Allied Personal Social Services*, Cmnd 3703. London: HMSO.

Seedhouse, D. (1986) *Health: The Foundations for Achievement*. Chichester: John Wiley.

Seedhouse, D. (1991) *Liberating Medicine*. Chichester: Wiley.

Segal, L. (1986) *The Dream of Reality: Heinz von Foerster's Constructivism*. New York: Norton.

Shemmings, D. and Thoburn, J. (1990) *Parental Participation in Child Protection Conferences*. Norwich: University of East Anglia.

Sheppard, M. (1991) *Mental Health Work in the Community*. London: Falmer Press.

Sheridan, C.L. and Radmacher, S.A. (1992) *Health Psychology: Challenging the Biomedical Model*. New York: John Wiley.

Shilling, C. (1993) *The Body and Social Theory*. London: Sage.

Shotter, J. (1986) Speaking practically: Whorf, the formative function of communication and knowing of the third kind, in L. Rosnow and M. Georgoudi (eds) *Contextualism and Understanding in Behavioural Science: Implications for Research and Theory*. New York: Praeger.

Shuchter, A. and Zisook, A. (1993) *Death and Dying*. Cambridge: Cambridge University Press.

Schutz, A. (1972) *The phenomenology of the social world*. (Translated by G. Walsh and F. Lerhnert. London: Heinemann.

Simpson, C.M., Simpson, R.J., Power, K.G., Salter, A. and Williams, G. (1994) GPs' and health visitors' participation in child protection case conferences, *Child Abuse Review*, 3: 211–30.

Smith, L. (1982) Models of nursing as the basis for curriculum development: Some rationales and implications, *Journal of Advanced Nursing*, 7: 117–27.

Smith, P. (1992) *The Emotional Labour of Nursing*. London: Macmillan.

Smithies, J. and Adams, L. (1993) Walking the tightrope: Issues in evaluation and community participation in *Health for All*, in J.K. Davies and M.P. Kelly (eds) *Healthy Cities: Research and Practice*. London: Routledge and Kegan Paul.

Sone, K. (1993) Mothers' help, *Community Care*, 962: 17.

Speechley, V. (1992) Patients as partners, *European Journal of Cancer Care*, 1: 22–5.

Speed, B. (1991) Reality exists OK? An argument against constructivism and social constructionism, *Family Therapy*, 13: 395–409.

Spielberger, C.D., Gorsuch, R.L., Lushene, R.E., Vagg, P.R. and Jacobs, G.A. (1983) *Manual for the State-Trait Anxiety Inventory*. Palo Alto, CA: Counselling Psychologists Press.

Spiers, J. (1994) NHS efficiency: The medieval knight stirs. Clinical effectiveness and better outcomes. The health summary, *The Briefing Paper for Policy Makers in Health*, X1: 5–7.

Stacey, M. (1988) *Sociology of Health and Healing*. London: Unwin Hyman.

Stainton Rogers, R. and Stainton Rogers, W. (1989) *Stories of Childhood: Shifting Agendas of Child Concern*. Hemel Hempstead: Harvester Wheatsheaf.

Stainton Rogers, W. (1991) *Explaining Health and Illness*. Hemel Hempstead: Harvester Wheatsheaf.

Stein, I.D. (1974) *Systems Theory, Science and Social Work*. Metuchen, NJ: Scarecrow.

Stephenson, E. (1964) Nursing service, education and research in a changing service, in J. Farndale (ed.) *Trends in the National Health Service*. Oxford: Pergamon Press.

Stevenson, C. (1994) On methods and methodology: A caucus race and being curious. Paper presented at the *Second London Conference on Closing the Gap Between Family Research and Family Therapy*, Institute of Psychiatry, London, March.

Stevenson, C. (1995a) Reflections on evaluating a course of family therapy, in J. Reed and S. Proctor (eds) *Practitioner Research in Health Care*. London: Chapman and Hall.

Stevenson, C. (1995b) Negotiating a therapeutic context. Unpublished PhD thesis, University of Northumbria.

Stoll, B. (ed.) (1991) *Social Dilemmas in Cancer Prevention*. London: Macmillan.

Stroebe, M.S., Stroebe, W. and Hansson, R.O. (1993) *Handbook of Bereavement: Research and Intervention*. Cambridge: Cambridge University Press.

Tannahill, A. (1985) What is health promotion? *Health Education Journal*, 49, 10–12.

Tattam, A. (1992) Complementary care to be law, *Nursing Times*, 88: 8.

Taylor, C., Roberts, J. and Dempster, H. (1993) Child sexual abuse: The child's perspective, in H. Ferguson, R. Gilligan and R. Torode (eds) *Surviving Childhood Adversity: Issues for Policy and Practice*. Dublin: Social Studies Press.

Taylor, S. and Godfrey, M. (1991) *Parental Involvement in Child Protection Case Conferences, and Evaluation of the Pilot Project*. North Tyneside: Social Services Department.

Thoburn, J., Lewis, A. and Shemmings, D. (1995) *Paternalism or Partnership? Family Involvement in the Child Protection Process*. London: HMSO.

Thomas, N. (1994) The social worker as bad object: A response to Marguerite Valentine, *British Journal of Social Work*, 24: 749–54.

Toseland, R.W., Palmer-Ganeless, J. and Chapman, D. (1986) Teamwork in psychiatric settings, *Social Work*, 3: 46–52.

Turner, B. (1984) *The Body and Society*. Oxford: Blackwell.

Turner, B. (1987) *Medical Power and Social Knowledge*. London: Sage.

Turner, B. (1992) *Regulating Bodies*. London: Routledge and Kegan Paul.

Twinn, S. and Cowley, S. (1992) *The Principles of Health Visiting: A Reexamination*. London: Health Visitors' Association and UK Standing Conference on Health Visitor Education.

UKCC (1992) *Code of Professional Conduct*. London: United Kingdom Central Council for Nursing and Midwifery.

Valentine, M. (1994) The social worker as 'bad object', *British Journal of Social Work*, 24: 71–88.

Vaughan, B. (1986) Knowing that and knowing how: The role of the lecturer practitioner, in B. Kershaw and J. Salvage (eds) *Models for Nursing*. London: Scutari.

Vetter, N., Jones, D. and Victor, C. (1986) Health visiting with the elderly in general practice, in A. While (ed.) *Research in Preventive Community Nursing Care*. Chichester: John Wiley.

Vickers, A. (1994) Use of complementary therapies, *British Medical Journal*, 309: 1161.

Waldby, C., Clancy, A., Emetchi, J. and Summerfield, C. for Dympna House (1989) Theoretical perspectives on father–daughter incest, in E. Driver and A. Droison (eds) *Child Sexual Abuse: Feminist Perspectives*. London: Macmillan.

Walters, K. (1990) Critical thinking and the Vulcanisation of students, *Journal of Higher Education*, 61: 448–67.

Wambach, J.A. (1985) The grief process as a social construct, *Omega*, 16: 201–11.

Watson, J. (1979) *Nursing: The Philosophy and Science of Caring*. Boston, MA: Little, Brown.

Watson, J. (1993) Male body image and health beliefs: A qualitative study and implications for health promotion practice, *Health Education Journal*, 52: 246–52.

Wattam, C. (1992) *Making a Case in Child Protection*. Harlow: Longman.

Watzlawick, P. (1976) *How Real is Real: Confusion, Disinformation, Communication. An Anecdotal Introduction to Communications Theory*. New York: Random House.

Watzlawick, P. (ed.) (1984) *The Invented Reality: How Do We Know What We Believe We Know?* New York: Norton.

Wear, A., French, R.K. and Lonie, I.M. (1985) *The Medical Renaissance of the Sixteenth Century*. Cambridge: Cambridge University Press.

Webb, C. (1984) Feminist methodology in nursing research, *Journal of Advanced Nursing*, 9: 248–56.

Webb, C. (1990) Nursing models in the curriculum, *Nurse Education Today*, 10: 299–306.

Webb, C. (1992) The use of the first person in academic writing: Objectivity, language and gate keeping, *Journal of Advanced Nursing*, 17: 747–52.

Webb, P. (1988) Living with cancer – complementary care, in R. Tiffany (ed.) *Oncology for Nurses and Health Care Professionals*. London: Harper Collins.

Weightman, K. (1988) Managing from below: Social work and child abuse, *Social Work Today*, 20: 16–17.

Weil, A. (1983) *Health and Healing*. Boston, MA: Houghton Mifflin.

Weiss, G.R. (1993) *Clinical Oncology*, International edn. Englewood Cliffs, NJ: Prentice Hall.

Wellings, K. (1988) Perceptions of risk – media treatments of AIDS, in P. Aggleton and H. Homans (eds) *Social Aspects of AIDS*. London: Falmer Press.

West, R. (1992) Alternative medicine: Prospects and speculations, in M. Saks (ed.) *Alternative Medicine in Britain*. Oxford: Oxford University Press.

Whitehead, A.N. and Russell, B. (1926) *Principia Mathematica*. Cambridge: Cambridge University Press.

Whitehead, M. (1987) *The Health Divide*. London: Health Education Council.

Whyte, W.F. (1984) *Learning from the Field: A Guide from Experience*. London: Sage.

Wilkinson, S. (1995) Aromatherapy and massage in palliative care, *International Journal of Palliative Nursing*, 1: 21–30.

Williams, C. (1993) Expert evidence in cases of child abuse, *Archives of Disease in Childhood*, 68: 712–14.

Williams, G. and Popay, J. (1994) Lay knowledge and the privilege of experience, in J. Gabe *et al.* (eds) *Challenging Medicine*. London: Routledge and Kegan Paul.

Williamson, J. (1981) Screening, surveillance and case finding, in T. Arie (ed.) *Health Care of the Elderly*. London: Croom Helm.

Wilson, E.O. (1975) *Sociobiology: The New Synthesis*. Cambridge, MA: Belknap.

Winter, R. (1989) *Learning from Experience: Principles and Practice in Action Research*. London: Falmer Press.

Wittgenstein, L. (1953) *Philosophical Investigations* (translated by G.E.M. Allscombe). Oxford: Blackwell.

Wolcock, I. and Horowitz, B. (1979) Child maltreatment and material deprivation among AFDC-recipient families, *Social Services Review*, 53: 175–94.

Worden, J.W. (1983) *Grief Counselling and Grief Therapy*. London: Tavistock/Routledge and Kegan Paul.

World Health Organization (1946) *Constitution*. New York: WHO.

World Health Organization (1978) Declaration of Alma-Ata, reproduced in *World Health*, August/September 1988, pp. 16–17.

World Health Organization (1984) *Health Promotion: A Discussion Document on the Concept and Principles*. Copenhagen: WHO Regional Office for Europe.

World Health Organization (1990) *Cancer Pain Relief and Palliative Care*. Geneva: WHO.

World Health Organization Study Group on Nursing Beyond the Year 2000 (1994) *Nursing beyond the Year 2000*. Geneva: WHO.

Yearwood-Dance, L. (1992) Use of relaxation in patients receiving radiation therapy to decrease symptom distress, in C.D. Bailey (ed.) *Cancer Nursing Changing Frontiers*. Proceedings of the Seventh International Conference on Cancer Nursing, Vienna. Oxford: Rapid Communications of Oxford.

Youngson, R.M. (1989) *Grief: Rebuilding Your Life after Bereavement*. Newton Abbot: David and Charles.

Yule, W. and Hemsley, D. (1977) Single case method in medical physiology, in S.J. Rachman (ed.) *Contributions to Medical Psychology*. Oxford: Pergamon Press.

Zola, I.K. (1977) Healthism and disabling medicalization, in I. Illich, I.K. Zola, J. McKnight, J. Caplan and H. Shaiken, *Disabling Professions*. London: Marion Boyars.

Index